Living with Grief: Cancer and End-of-Life Care

Edited by
Kenneth J. Doka & Amy S. Tucci
Foreword by Perry G. Fine

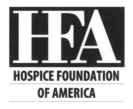

**HOSPICE FOUNDATION
OF AMERICA**

This book is part of Hospice Foundation of America's *Living with Grief*® series.

© 2010 Hospice Foundation of America®

This book is part of HFA's *Living with Grief*® series.

Ordering information:

Call Hospice Foundation of America: 800-854-3402

Or write:
Hospice Foundation of America
1710 Rhode Island Avenue, NW #400
Washington, DC 20036

Or visit HFA's Web site:
www.hospicefoundation.org

Assistant Editor: Keith Johnson
Layout and Design: The YGS Group
Cover Illustration: Delaine Driscoll at The Children's Room Center for Grieving Children in Arlington Massachusetts

Publisher's Cataloging-in-Publication
(Provided by Quality Books, Inc.)

Living with grief : cancer and end-of-life care / edited by
   Kenneth J. Doka & Amy S. Tucci ; foreword by Perry Fine.
      p. cm.
      Includes bibliographical references and index.
      LCCN 2009943099
      ISBN-13: 978-1-893349-11-7
      ISBN-10: 1-893349-11-X

         1. Grief. 2. Bereavement--Psychological aspects.
      3. Loss (Psychology) 4. Cancer--Patients. 5. Terminal
      care. 6. Palliative treatment.   I. Doka, Kenneth J.
      II. Tucci, Amy S.

   BF575.G7L58 2010   155.9'37
                                 QBI09-600232

Dedication

To my four lifelong friends
For being part of my life—through childhood and adolescence—still there

Elizabeth Galindo
Larry Laterza
Lynn Vigliotti-Miller
Eric Schwarz

And to Kathleen Dillon
A special companion through many adult years

Kenneth J. Doka

For Cecil McCullars and Frank Tucci

Amy S. Tucci

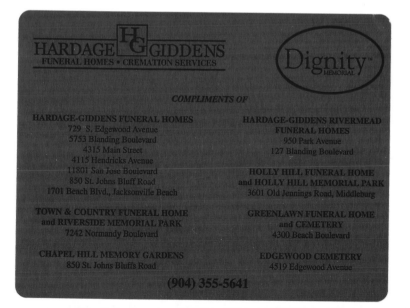

Contents

Foreword
Perry G. Fine i

Acknowledgments..v

PART I:
THE NATURE OF CANCER...1

1. **Cancer: An Historical and Cultural Perspective**
   Kenneth J. Doka...3

2. **Cancer and the History of Hospice**
   Stephen R. Connor 13

3. **Difficult Choices: Making Decisions When Cure Is Not Possible**
   Stuart Farber 25

4. **After the Battle, Journeys with Cancer: Changing Metaphors of Illness**
   Neil Small...39

PART II:
TREATING CANCER 53

5. **Treatment Options in Cancer**
   Brad Stuart 55

6. **Complementary and Alternative Cancer Therapies:**
   Don't Ask, Don't Tell
   Lynda Shand...67

7. **Ethical Dilemmas in the Treatment of Cancer**
   Nancy Berlinger and Bruce Jennings 83

8. **The Transition to Palliative Care**
   Brad Stuart 97

9. **End-Stage Cancer: The Role of Palliative Care and Hospice**
   Sherry R. Schachter 109

Part III:
Psychosocial Aspects of Cancer Care..............................123

10. **Guilt and Self-Blame: Coping with Cancer Causation**
Kenneth A. Krajewski, Erin S. Costanzo, Matthew D. LoConte, and
Noelle K. LoConte..125

11. **Cancer in Children and Adolescents: Psychosocial Dimensions**
Marianne Walsh...137

 Personal Perspective: Vivienne's Story
 Mary Martin..147

12. **Facing Cancer: The Gender Dimension**
Neil Thompson...151

Part IV:
Grief and Cancer...163

 Personal Perspective: He Was Still Our Child
 Karl Snepp..165

13. **Cancer, Anticipatory Grief, and Anticipatory Mourning**
Charles A. Corr...169

14. **Grief After a Death From Cancer**
Kenneth J. Doka...181

 Personal Perspective: Antonia's Story
 Yvette Colón...195

Index 201

Foreword

Dr. Perry G. Fine

"If not you, then who?" These words were spoken to me by a wise and deeply concerned mentor during a time of extreme doubt that I was experiencing as a medical intern. I was wondering whether I had anything of value at all to offer the patients under my care who were dying from far-advanced cancer. This simple but profound rhetorical rejoinder to my expressed sense of inadequacy turned me on my heel, actually and metaphorically, to return and attend to my patients as they lay dying, with conviction no longer to be demoralized by a lack of ability to prescribe a cure, but rather to be motivated to help reduce the burden imposed by their disease.

Several years later, and seemingly a world apart from that linoleum-lined county hospital, I was sitting in an oak and gilded boardroom of a prestigious cancer center at a meeting to discuss cancer care. Upper echelon directors of the center were proudly reviewing the latest data demonstrating small, but notable increases in 5-year survival rates for patients with certain solid tumors treated there. Ebullience and congratulations were plentiful, until someone asked: "What happens to the other 48.3% of patients who don't live 5 years, and the ones who live longer than 5 years, but still succumb to their disease?" Whatever the opposite of "ebullience" is, it was, at that moment, positively palpable. A stunned silence gave way to a deftly managed change in subject by our host, and the conversation meandered elsewhere. No one dared allude to, no less mention, the "d" word again.

More than 30 years have passed since I witnessed my first cancer death as a healthcare worker. Yes, wonderful progress in the treatment of several malignancies has occurred, but metastatic disease still takes a terrible toll. I am still haunted by the images of that first experience and the many more that followed. It is not the physical ravages of this terrible group of diseases we subsume under the singular and terrifying term "cancer" that makes me shiver as I conjure up these memories. I was amply prepared for the sights, the smells, the sounds of cancer; although not easy to get used to, we quickly adapt and we also learn quite effectively *to pretend* not to be bothered. We learn to parry the worst of what disease and trauma bring so that we can get past the revulsion and do what needs to be done. The latent images that refuse to be extinguished in my mind's eye is that pathognomonic look of desperate loneliness embedded in the actual eyes of those patients as they lay dying—

that, and more so, the realization that we unintentionally but no less actually contribute to it. We come and go, perform our duties, but we rarely *connect*, and it is connection that is so desperately needed. Our methods change, protocols become updated, but outside of hospice and palliative care settings, that outcome largely remains the same. We are taught to effectively manage our own horror by mastering the treatment imperative: focus on the disease; fight the disease. And, even in the face of overwhelmingly irrefutable evidence of progressive and irreversible disease, we promote the delusion of cure and equate this misdirected posturing as "hope."

Early on, before cancer has spread, these warrior-like devices and noble aspirations may have great value and virtue. But in far-advanced metastatic cancer, the seemingly polar but equally fearsome forms of neglect, consisting of either highly aggressive and persistent "anti-cancer" treatment or "I have nothing further to offer" dismissiveness, are nothing more or less than cynicisms disguised as expertise. William Osler recognized this temptation when he stated, "To accept a great group of maladies, against which we have never had and can scarcely ever hope to have curative measures, makes some men as sensitive as though we were ourselves responsible for their existence. These very cases are 'rocks of offence' to many good fellows whose moral decline dates from the rash promise to cure. We work by wit and not by witchcraft, and while patients have our tenderest care, and we must do what is best for the relief of their sufferings, we should not bring the art of medicine into disrepute by quack-like promises to heal, or by wire-drawn attempts at cure, adding continuate and inexorable maladies."

The misapprehension that acknowledging mortality, even imminent death, is somehow tantamount to acquiescing to disease, or inviting a premature death, opens the door to excessive suffering on one or both of these two all-too-common fronts: burdensome, and even torturous, treatments without likely therapeutic benefit, and abandonment. Grief can take a terrible toll, and the denial of death—as vibrant a cultural norm today as it was when the book of the same name was written a generation ago—fuels and protracts the paralyzing response to loss. In that seminal work, Ernest Becker observes: "As long as man is an ambiguous creature he can never banish anxiety; what he can do instead is to use anxiety as an eternal spring for growth into new dimensions of thought and trust." And so, this book has been prepared. By confronting, amassing, and finally organizing their own "anxieties" into this series of essays, this group of extraordinarily insightful healthcare professionals provides us with a great gift in that we may better serve those patients and their families as they face the ultimate loss. By provoking "thought and trust," and thereby redefining hope in the most sanguine of ways, these essays help us to connect with patients and families at their time of ultimate loss without losing ourselves in the process. In so doing, they provide the answer to the question that must be continually asked and answered: "If not you, then who?"

Perry G. Fine, MD, is a professor of anesthesiology in the Pain Research Center, School of Medicine at the University of Utah in Salt Lake City. Fine currently chairs the National Initiative on Pain Control and serves on the boards of directors of the American Academy of Pain Medicine, the Society for Arts in Healthcare, and the American Pain Foundation. His most recent book is The Hospice Companion: Best Practices for Interdisciplinary Assessment and Care of Common Problems During the Last Phase of Life.

REFERENCES

Becker, E. (1973). *The denial of death* (p. 92). New York: The Free Press.

Osler, W. (1909). The treatment of disease. *Canada Lancet, 42,* 899–912.

Acknowledgments

We always find the acknowledgments a pleasure to write. It is a joy to recognize each year the individuals in our lives who provide both personal and professional support. It is an amazing feat that the Hospice Foundation of America can annually produce a book in addition to, and as part of, an annual teleconference. This is so much due to the heroic efforts of the HFA staff, past and present. Included here are David Abrams, Lisa McGahey Veglahn, Sophie Viteri Berman, Keith Johnson, Kristen Baker, Susan Belsinger, Marcia Eaker, Marceline Bateky, Chester Velasco, and Krista Renenger. Myra McPherson, a board member, contributed in her special way to this year's book development. And, of course, we acknowledge all the authors who share their stories and knowledge.

Each year as the process of putting this annual book together comes to a close, I remember how a former staff member summed up the Hospice Foundation of America after a particularly long day. She said, "You know what we are? We're the Little Engine that Could." Those familiar with the fantastic children's book of the same title will appreciate her metaphor. Those who really know HFA will appreciate it even more. We are, unlike our grand name implies, a small foundation with a tiny staff and a dedication to try our hardest to advance professional knowledge and consumer awareness of hospice care and bereavement. And more often than we would probably like, as we approach various projects before us, HFA's staff (and that includes Ken Doka, who is not actually a staff member, but he works like a full-time employee) is surely thinking as the little engine did, "I think I can, I think I can." So, with admiration for the relentless energy, dedication, and enthusiasm he contributes to HFA, I thank Ken Doka, my coeditor, for his vision and leadership on yet another *Living with Grief* book. I also thank Keith Johnson, managing editor, for his sensibilities and sensitivities when it comes to editing a book with a potentially overwhelming subject as *Cancer and End-of-Life Care*. Keith shares the value that we at HFA consider most important: delivering a quality product that has the potential to help advance the mission of hospice care. On a personal note, I would like to thank my family for their support of my work at HFA and the insights that they each provide. It is with some embarrassment that I disclose that it was a family member's idea to address the issue of cancer. We didn't have to agree, of course, but when we started exploring Cancer and End-of-Life Care as a potential topic for 2010, we knew she was right about it, even at age 12. Cancer seems to touch us all.

—Amy S. Tucci

It is always a joy to work with Amy. She brings to the process sharp editorial skills, grounded insights, and a deep sense of commitment to mission and quality.

There are so many family and friends that I need to thank. My son and daughter-in-law, Michael and Angelina, and my grandchildren, Kenny and Lucy, provide love and insist upon balance. My godchildren—James Rainbolt, Scott Carlson, Christine Romano, and Keith Whitehead (and their families)— remain important even in their adulthood. Kathy Dillon, my sister, Dorothy and my brother, Franky, and all of their families as well as Dylan Rieger, Ellie Andersen, Jim, Karen and Greg Cassa, Linda and Russell Tellier, Jill Boyer, Lynn Miller, and Tom and Lorraine Carlson are always there when I need them. Three lifelong friends, Larry Laterza, Lynn Miller, and Eric Schwarz, were recognized in the Dedication. And I am blessed with good neighbors including Paul Kimbal, Carol Ford, Allen and Gail Greenstein, Jim and Mary Millar, Robert and Tracey Levy, Fred and Lisa Amore, and Chris and Dorotta Fields.

Colleagues at the College of New Rochelle, the Association of Death Education and Counseling (ADEC), and The International Work Group on Dying, Death, and Bereavement (IWG) provide stimulation and friendship. I also wish to thank my administrators and staff at the College of New Rochelle for providing the support and freedom that encourages my work. Here I acknowledge President Stephen Sweeny, President-Elect Judith Huntington, Vice President Dorothy Escribano, Dean Marie Ribarich, and Program Director Wendi Vescio, as well as the ongoing support offered by Diane Lewis and Vera Mezzaucella.

As always, we acknowledge the continuing legacy of the late Jack Gordon, founder and former chair of the Hospice Foundation of America.

—Kenneth J. Doka

The Nature of Cancer

Cancer is not a single disease but, rather, more than 150 distinct diseases, classified into four major groupings. *Carcinomas*, the most common form of cancer, affect the skin and skin-like tissues of the internal organs. *Sarcomas* attack bones, muscles, cartilage, fat, and linings of the lungs, abdomen, heart, central nervous system, and blood vessels. There are also *leukemias* that develop in blood, bone marrow, and the spleen, and *lymphomas*, or cancers that emerge in the lymphatic system.

Over the past decades, there has been considerable success in treating some, albeit not all, forms of cancer. Prevention efforts, early detection and diagnosis, as well as advances in treatment, have played a role in this success.

Yet despite the success, people still die of cancer—over 500,000 Americans in 2008. Cancer is the second greatest killer in the U.S., behind heart disease. Because of these statistics, there is a need to review the particular issues that emerge when dealing with cancer and end-of-life care—for patients, for families and intimate networks, and for health professionals.

Kenneth Doka begins this section by exploring the history of cancer. He notes the historical paradox of cancer: It is both an old and new disease. Cancer existed in antiquity but emerged as a leading cause of death in the Industrial Age, partly because of lengthened life spans and increased carcinogenic exposure. Doka notes another paradox as well. In order to increase the governmental role in treating cancer, advocates needed to build a fear of cancer while maintaining a sense of hope that treatment could one day effectively end cancer's threat.

Stephen Connor explores another aspect of cancer history: the role of hospice in cancer treatment. As he notes, hospice was originally developed to treat cancer. For the most part, cancer had a relatively predictable trajectory that made it easier to demarcate between curative and palliative modes of treatment. In addition, cancer patients needed ongoing rather than intermittent care. Many of the hospice breakthroughs in pain and symptom management were developed in response to cancer. The challenge for hospice and palliative care is now to adapt the model for other diseases since cancer patients are no longer the exclusive focus of hospice care.

While Connor addresses the history of hospice and palliative care, Stuart Farber addresses it on a personal level. How does someone make the decision to seek hospice or palliative care and forgo curative or life-extending treatment? To Farber, these are collaborative decisions, made in a context of honest and frank conversation that allows medical staff, families, and patients to fully understand options and goals of treatment.

Neil Small continues this theme, ending this section. To Small, metaphoric understanding is a large part of the process of narrative: the ways we make meaning of the world. Building upon (but significantly diverting from) the early work of Susan Sontag (1978, 1989), Small contends that cancer evokes a multiplicity of metaphors. Some of these are clearly militaristic. We need to *fight* cancer, not *give up*. We wage war against cancer. Such metaphors are counter to the hospice model of care. After all, is it not more heroic to fight to the bitter end, going down in a blaze of glory? But Small reminds us of another metaphor: *journey*. Cancer patients *travel a path* or *climb a mountain*. The image of a journey suggests a beginning and a direction of travel. It is the role of hospice to help patients and families navigate the rough terrain as the journey through cancer comes to an end.

REFERENCES

Sontag, S. (1978). *Illness as metaphor.* New York: McGraw-Hill.

Sontag, S. (1989). *AIDS and its metaphors.* New York: Farrar, Straus & Giroux.

Cancer: An Historical and Cultural Perspective

Kenneth J. Doka

C ancer is both an ancient and modern disease. Identified and named in antiquity, yet it remains a scourge of more developed societies. Its origins, Sorkin (2009) hypothesizes, might lie in the very control mechanisms that arose early in evolution as individual cells began to come together in multicellular communities. To Sorkin, this allowed the evolutionary advantage of specialization and increasing complexity. However, it would necessitate a biological mechanism that would control the reproduction of these now specialized cells. Sorkin suggests that cancer emerges when this control mechanism fails.

Cancer was clearly evident early in history. Egyptian mummies offer evidence of osteosarcoma (bone cancer). The two earliest medical documents, the Edwin Smith papyrus (ca. 1600 BC) and the Ebers papyrus (ca. 1550 BC), both describe it. Hippocrates, often considered the father of medicine, was the first to name it *carcinos* and *carcinoma*—names that the Roman physician Celsus, three centuries later, translated into the Latin equivalent *cancer*, for crab. It is open to conjecture as to why Hippocrates named the disease after the crab. It may have referred to the crab-like shape of tumors he observed, the similarity of the pain to a crab bite, or perhaps to the tenacity of the disease's spread. Later, Galen, another prominent Roman physician, used the term *oncos* (a root for the term *oncology*), from the Greek term for swelling, to describe these cancerous tumors (Olson, 1989).

While cancer's roots are ancient, it is in many ways a disease of development. It is a disease of both an aging society and an industrial economy. Only with a requisite level of development can the population reach an age to be more likely to contract cancer. Only with a society that is able to eradicate many acute diseases and control epidemics can populations survive to develop cancer. Medical care has to be at a level that can recognize and diagnose cancer. Industrialized societies also provide the diets, habits, and exposures to carcinogenic chemicals and pollutants that increase the risk and rates of cancer.

In the United States, those conditions were not fully in place until the late 19th century. At that time, the death rates from cancer began to increase. However, there was still one event beyond these rising rates that would focus attention on this emerging illness. Just as Rock Hudson's death and Magic Johnson's diagnosis of HIV infection increased public awareness of AIDS, the copious and melodramatic press accounts of former President Grant's battle with throat cancer and his death in 1885 galvanized public attention on cancer (Patterson, 1987). The American population was then well aware of cancer and deeply dreaded the disease, causing a sense of fear and shame superseded in more contemporary times only by AIDS.

HISTORICAL PERSPECTIVES ON CANCER CAUSATION, TREATMENT, AND PREVENTION

Causation

Cancer is a complex disease or, in reality, a set of more than 150 distinct diseases. This complexity confounded understandings of causation, treatment, and prevention. In the prescientific era, causation was generally viewed as the result of a curse, the will of God, Karma, or the nature of fate. However the earliest developed medical histories did attempt to account for cancer. One of the earliest medical theories was Hippocrates's humoral theory. Hippocrates suggested that the body contained four basic humors, or body fluids: blood, phlegm, black bile, and yellow bile. Any imbalance of these humors caused illness. Cancer thus was caused by an excess of black bile in a given area or part of the body. Hippocrates's work was well accepted until the Renaissance. Then other theories emerged suggesting cancer was caused by degenerating lymph, irritation, proposed cellular material labeled *blastema* that arose from normal tissue, or even from parasites—an idea that won a Nobel prize in 1926 (Olson, 1989).

It was basic scientific work that began to unlock the secret of cancer. Rudolph Virchow, the father of cellular theory, demonstrated that cancer cells derived from other cells in the body. Watson and Crick, in discovering the chemical structure of DNA, created a basis for contemporary understandings of cancer causation. This allowed the identification of *oncogenes*, or mutated genes that cause cells to grow uncontrollably, and tumor suppressor genes that slow cell division, eliminate cells, and repair DNA errors. We now understand that a range of factors—including chemicals, radiation, viruses, and genetic factors—can stimulate oncogenes and inhibit tumor suppressor genes, leading to cancer.

Treatment

The earliest references to cancer note treatment from a *fire drill*—a likely reference to attempts to cauterize the tumor (Olson, 1989). However, even in the Edwin Smith papyrus, the pessimism that still surrounds cancer was evident. There was, the document confirms, no treatment. Both Hippocrates and Galen concurred that the disease was incurable.

However, Galen recognized the possibility that the total surgical removal of the tumor could cure breast cancer, provided the disease had not spread. Unfortunately, the early state of surgery—without anesthesia or antiseptics—often brought death as an inevitable complication of surgical treatment. However, with the development of anesthesia in 1846, cancer surgery could begin to progress. Conscious of the fact that tumors tended to spread, pioneer cancer surgeons such as Bilroth, Halstead, and Hanley suggested that the entire tumor be removed as well as any lymph glands in the area where the tumor was located. These extensive operations often resulted in amputations and mutilation that made cancer surgery as feared as the disease.

Stephen Paget, an English surgeon, advanced the understanding of the process of metastasis, or the spread of cancer. Paget hypothesized that cancer cells were carried throughout the bloodstream but would only grow in certain organs, much like seeds could only grow in compatible soil. This understanding, later confirmed by advances in cellular and molecular biology, allowed a more specialized approach that combined less invasive surgery with other approaches such as radiation therapy, hormonal therapy, and chemotherapy. Recently, additional approaches such as ultrasound, magnetic resonance imaging (MRI), positron emission tomography (PET) scans, and computed tomography (CT) have minimized the need for exploratory therapy. Other techniques such as endoscopy, laparoscopic surgery, and thorascopic surgery allow the removal of tumors through tubes inserted through body orifices or openings created by small incisions, further minimizing the need for invasive procedures. In addition, cyrotherapy, lasers, and radiofrequency ablation use extreme cold or heat to destroy cancer cells, and hold promise for future surgical treatment.

In addition to surgery, other therapies also were developed to treat cancer. In 1896, a German physicist, Wilhelm Roentgen, discovered the X-ray. Within

3 years, X-rays were being used for both diagnosis and cancer treatment. However, it was soon realized that the X-rays could both cure and cause cancer: many radiologists used their own arms to test the strength of the ray, and some of them later developed leukemia. As with surgery, the challenge has been to focus the X-ray on the cancerous cells while trying to avoid radiating healthy cells. Technological developments have allowed more carefully focused X-rays and use of chemical modifiers that make cancer cells more sensitive to radiation.

Chemotherapy began later. During World War II, army scientists, trying to develop protective methods against mustard gas, discovered that the compound nitrogen mustard could kill cancer cells by damaging the DNA of such cells. Soon other drugs were found that could interfere with the replication and growth of cancer cells. Chemotherapy has been found to be an effective cure for some forms of cancer as well as a way to control the disease, extending life when cure is not possible. Moreover, chemotherapy has been used in adjuvant therapy, that is, in combination with surgery and/or radiation to kill cancer cells that might have spread beyond a localized area.

As with other approaches such as radiation and surgery, the objective of chemotherapy is to kill cancer cells with the least possible damage to other cells or other problematic side effects. For this reason, there is continued development of use of multiple chemotherapeutic agents; new ways to deliver drugs, such as liposomal therapy (which delivers chemotherapy inside liposomes, a fatty coating, to both decrease side effects and better target medications); and other techniques to target chemotherapy or to enhance the immune system and augment normal biological functions to resist cancers.

The treatment of cancer has been an incredible success story given the centuries that the disease was considered inevitably fatal. In many ways, that success was due to an unusual partnership between medicine and government—itself a testimony to the efforts of the American Society for Control of Cancer, renamed in 1944 as the American Cancer Society. Under the leadership of Clarence Cook Little, the American Society for Control of Cancer mobilized women's clubs and the media to encourage the federal government to take an unprecedented role in funding cancer research. This effort led to both the establishment of cancer control as the number one health initiative and the development of the National Cancer Institute. This success was the result of the confluence of a number of factors. First, the New Deal administration had an activist view of government. Second, the American

Society for Control of Cancer had a carefully nuanced message. Part stressed fear: Cancer could strike anyone at any time. Yet, the fear was tempered with a sense of optimism: Cancer could be treated, possibly even cured; funds would not be wasted. Finally, the American Society for Control of Cancer was able to unify—with the possible exclusion of some unorthodox clinicians, medical researchers, and patient and family groups—major organizations in cancer research and advocacy and other stakeholders such as pharmaceutical companies in one common cause (Doka, 1997).

Cancer has remained a major health priority, so much so that in 1971, then-President Richard Nixon declared "war on cancer." This resulted in the National Cancer Act of 1971, which increased funding for cancer research and gave the National Cancer Institute special autonomy within the National Institutes of Health. Even now there is a Senate bill—the 21st Century Cancer Access to Life-Saving Early Detection, Research, and Treatment (ALERT) Act, introduced by Senators Kennedy and Hutchison—that seeks to increase funding for early detection and treatment. Despite these considerable efforts, success is mixed. While cancer remains a major source of mortality, there have been declines in cancer deaths for all age groups, with younger populations benefitting most. Moreover, the rates are uneven. There has been great success in treating certain cancers such as lymphoma and leukemia, while other cancers such as lung cancer remain resistant (Kort, Paneth, & Vande Woude, 2009).

Despite this progress, the fear of cancer and the limitations of conventional treatment for so much of cancer's history enabled cancer quackery to flourish. Numerous substances were claimed to control or cure cancer, and looking at a few examples of some of the more contemporary cancer hoaxes is illustrative. In the 1940s, Dr. William F. Koch sold highly distilled water that he claimed held a 1-trillionth part of the chemical glyoxylide. More than 3,000 people paid anywhere from $25 to $300 for this useless drug. Koch was tried twice, but one trial ended in a mistrial and the other resulted in a hung jury. Koch soon retired to Brazil, but the Koch treatment was still offered in Mexico.

Harry Hoxsey soon filled the gap left by Koch. Hoxsey claimed that he had a formula for two medications that his great grandfather found more than 100 years earlier. The two medications consisted of a variety of extracts as well as lactated papsin and potassium iodide, none of which had any proven ability to treat cancer. His Dallas-based clinic offered a lifetime supply of the drug for $400. Hoxsey used his funds, and those of his oil investments, to fight government attempts to shut down his clinic. The Food and Drug Administration finally succeeded in 1960 after patients had spent in excess of $50 million for this useless treatment. Soon other useless treatments such as Krebiozen and the Rand vaccine were offered, again despite the lack of any medical evidence that such procedures helped. In fact, the Rand vaccine was shown to be not only bacterially contaminated, but possibly carcinogenic (Cassileth, Lusk, Strouse, & Bodenheimer, 1984). Federal laws to regulate drug safety and prevent false claims originally arose from attempts to eliminate these false claims to cure cancer.

Even today there still exists a significant cancer underground. This underground offers alternative and unverified treatments for cancer, such as amygdalin and laetrile, suggesting that the "cancer establishment," beholden to the pharmaceutical industry, is involved in a conspiracy to withhold inexpensive and unobtrusive treatments from the public. Alternative treatments that are used instead of conventional treatments should be differentiated from complementary therapies such as nutritional regimens or guided imagery that are used along with conventional medical treatment.

Prevention

Cancer prevention has, along with treatment, been a major initiative in cancer efforts. Already in the 18th century, observers were noting factors that seemed to be associated with cancer. In 1713, an Italian physician, Bernardino Ramazzini, wondered if the very low rate of cervical cancer in nuns had some relationship to their celibacy. Fewer than 50 years later, in 1761, Dr. John Hill suggested that the new habit of snuffing tobacco might be causing an increase in cancers of the nose. Soon after, Dr. Percival Pott noted the high incidences of scrotum cancer in chimney sweeps. Since that time, the World Health Organization has noted more than 100 chemical, physical, and biological carcinogens, including viruses, that seem to increase risks for certain forms of cancer.

These epidemiological observations and later epidemiological studies have had two implications. First, they have led to considerable efforts to prevent cancer. For example, Pott's advocacy led to a number of attempts to regulate chimney sweeps, including age and sanitary requirements (e.g., a weekly bath, whether needed or not). In the United States, various attempts at prevention have included controlling exposure to radiation and other carcinogenic substances in air, water, or the environment, as well as numerous attempts to regulate tobacco use. A second implication has been less desirable: the rise of a culture that potentially blames victims for participating in activities, such as smoking, that increase risk.

A Brief Note on Cancer and Culture

Since cancer risk is due to the interaction of biological and environmental factors, it is unsurprising that there are significant differences in rates of cancer incidence and mortality among cultures and cultural groups within a country. As stated earlier, cancer itself, while universal and ancient, tends to be more prevalent in developed countries. Differences in incidence and mortality may reflect ethnic differences in exposure to carcinogenic elements, such as the hepatitis C virus, or other risk factors evident in diet or behaviors, such as tobacco usage. However these differences in cancer incidence and mortality also may reflect differences in awareness of symptoms of certain cancers or differences in access to early screening or appropriate treatment. In other cases, certain cultural groups may delay seeking health care due to the initial use of traditional treatments or perceived stigma associated with cancer diagnosis (Boston, 2007).

Reducing cultural disparities within the United States or other multiethnic nations will likely involve a number of strategies. Research has reaffirmed that reducing inequalities in access and treatment does much to eliminate differences in mortality (Cooper, Smaje, & Arber, 1998). Culturally appropriate education efforts, especially in the language of targeted groups, are also useful. In addition, health professionals should be educated in the meanings that cancer has in the cultures they regularly treat. As Boston (2007) notes, such education can enhance communication and collaborations among health professionals, families, and patients.

Conclusion

Throughout the 20th century, there has been considerable, albeit uneven, progress on cancer. In that time, the nature of cancer has been better understood, and there have been significant successes in treatment and prevention. This century promises even more. The human genome project may improve the understanding of cancer. Newer therapeutic approaches—including targeted therapies, adjuvant therapy, and strategies designed to enhance immune systems—offer promise of continued advances in treatment.

While one aspect of the history of cancer has been progress in detecting and treating the disease, another facet of cancer's history has been the great fear that cancer generates. Cancer has been one of a number of diseases that have been dreaded throughout history. Some, such as the horrific Black Plague, have created fear because of their sudden devastation—killing tens of thousands in a great epidemic. However, there is another type of dreaded disease, feared not for the rapidity by which they devastate communities, but rather for the slow way that victims die. They are disfiguring and dehabilitating, chronic and terminal. These diseases have included tuberculosis, leprosy, syphilis, and cancer (Doka, 1997). The fear of these diseases provoked a search for a reason for disease—and that search often resulted in blaming the victim. The result was that the disease conferred stigma on the victim, adding isolation and shame to the burdens of illness.

To some degree, the stigma of cancer, at least in the United States, has lessened. In some ways this began in the 1940s as a survivor literature began to emerge that recounted the memoirs of persons that had survived cancer. The moral of these books was twofold: to emphasize the importance of early detection and treatment, and to minimize the stigma victims experienced. To some extent it has been successful; cancer is no longer whispered and hidden. Yet some forms of cancer still retain a sense of blame and stigma. While men can be diagnosed with breast cancer, most share the diagnosis with only a few friends. Colon cancer, still a major killer, provokes questions of whether the victim regularly had colonoscopies. If not, the victim may be perceived as self-negligent.

Lung cancer remains highly stigmatizing, often carrying a sense of blame that lifestyle habits such as smoking caused the disease. In fact, recent restrictions on second-hand smoke further confer that sense of blame, affirming that the smoker is not only endangering self but others as well. Patterson (1987) notes that such restrictions gained ground only after the middle class began to cease smoking. In some ways the language associated with lung cancer—especially ads by the antismoking lobby that even if you choose to kill yourself by continuing to smoke, you must be prohibited from killing others by second-hand smoke—mimics the language of AIDS that described pediatric patients as the "innocent" victims of the disease, thereby implying another group is not so innocent.

Perhaps one of the next great advances in the struggle against cancer will be that even as one becomes aware of the complex interplay of biological, environmental, and behavioral factors that influence the incidence, treatment, and mortality rates of cancer, there is an affirmation that the focus of efforts remains to treat cancer patients humanely. Any blame should be on a cellular process gone awry—not the individual with the illness.

Kenneth J. Doka, PhD, *is a professor of gerontology at the Graduate School of the College of New Rochelle and senior consultant to the Hospice Foundation of America. A prolific editor and author, Dr. Doka's books include* Living with Grief: Diversity and End-of-Life Care; Living with Grief: Children and Adolescents; Living with Grief: Before and After Death; Death, Dying and Bereavement: Major Themes in Health and Social Welfare; Living with Grief: Ethical Dilemmas at the End of Life; Living with Grief: Alzheimer's Disease; Men Don't Cry, Women Do: Transcending Gender Stereotypes of Grief; Living with Grief: Loss in Later Life; Disenfranchised Grief: Recognizing Hidden Sorrow; Children Mourning, Mourning Children; Death and Spirituality; Living with Grief: After Sudden Loss; Living with Grief: When Illness Is Prolonged; Living with Grief: Who We Are, How We Grieve; Living with Grief: At Work, School and Worship; Caregiving and Loss: Family Needs, Professional Responses; AIDS, Fear and Society; Aging and Developmental Disabilities; *and* Disenfranchised Grief: New Directions, Challenges, and Strategies for Practice. *In addition, Dr. Doka has published more than 60 articles and book chapters. Dr. Doka is editor of* Omega *and* Journeys: A Newsletter to Help in Bereavement.

REFERENCES

Boston, P. (2007). Culture and cancer: The relevance of cultural orientation within cancer education programmes. *European Journal of Cancer Care, 2,* 72–76.

Cassileth, B. R., Lusk, E. J., Strouse, T. B., & Bodenheimer, B. J. (1984). Contemporary unorthodox treatments in cancer medicine: A study of patients, treatments, and practitioners. *Annals of Internal Medicine, 101,* 105–112.

Cooper, H., Smaje, C., & Arber, S. (1998). Use of health services by children and young people according to ethnicity and social class: Secondary analysis of a national survey. *British Journal of Medicine, 317,* 1047–1051.

Doka, K. J. (1997). *AIDS, fear, and society: Challenging the dreaded disease.* Philadelphia: Taylor & Francis.

Kort, E. J., Paneth, N., & Vande Woude, G. F. (2009). The decline in U.S. cancer mortality in people born since 1925. *Cancer Research, 69,* 6500–6505.

Olson, J. (1989). *The history of cancer: An annotated bibliography.* New York: Greenwood Press.

Patterson, J. T. (1987). *The dread disease: Cancer and modern American culture.* Cambridge, MA: Harvard University Press.

Sorkin, R. D. (2009). A historical perspective on cancer. Archived at http://www.physics.syr.edu/~sorkin/some.papers/128.cancer.pdf

CHAPTER

Cancer and the History of Hospice

Stephen R. Connor

In many respects, the way hospice care developed around the world has been influenced by the trajectory of cancer. Advanced malignant disease has a generally more predictable course than most other chronic conditions. Consequently, it is somewhat easier to identify patients who are believed to be near the end of life. The provision of hospice care as an ongoing, rather than intermittent, form of care delivery also is more consistent with the needs of cancer patients. Increasingly, however, those needing hospice and palliative care have noncancer diagnoses.

This chapter examines the history of hospice care and how that history was influenced by the needs of cancer patients, who initially were the primary target population. Also covered are the challenges of improving the accuracy of prognostication, the impact that increasing numbers of noncancer patients are having on the design and delivery of hospice care, and what that means for the future of hospice.

HISTORY OF MODERN HOSPICE CARE

The Irish Sisters of Charity founded Our Lady's Hospice for care of the dying in Dublin, and in 1900 they started a convent in London's East End. They visited the sick and dying in their homes. In 1902 they founded St. Joseph's Hospice for the dying poor in London. It was at St. Joseph's 50 years later that Dr. Cicely Saunders came to work and began to develop her approach to managing pain and the total needs of dying patients.

Modern hospice care began at St. Christopher's Hospice in Sydenham outside London in 1967. In the beginning of care at St. Christopher's, the patients were almost exclusively diagnosed with cancers. There might have been an occasional patient with a progressive life-limiting illness like amyotrophic lateral sclerosis (ALS), but the hospice focused on patients with advanced cancers.

Given that hospices in most countries began as charitable organizations with limited resources, hospice pioneers felt that those who could benefit most

13

were oncology patients who had significant pain and other symptoms that palliative care could more readily address. Until the late 1990s, Dr. Saunders did not favor provision of hospice care to most noncancer patients because she felt that there were other specialists better prepared to manage the symptoms and trajectories of patients with various forms of solid organ failure, including heart, lung, liver, kidney, and so forth (Connor, 1995).

Cancer and the Hospice Care Model

Modern hospice care began in the United Kingdom as an inpatient care model. Patients with cancer were admitted, usually in severe distress at advanced stages of illness, often near death. They could be transferred from home or commonly from other facilities that lacked the skills to effectively manage their symptoms. Over time, hospice professionals gained skill in effectively managing pain and other cancer symptoms, including nausea and vomiting, constipation, shortness of breath, skin breakdown, confusion and agitation, and so forth.

The effective use of opioids with cancer patients was a breakthrough in managing pain, the most troubling symptom of advanced cancer. Patients who seemed near death would undergo major improvement when their pain was controlled with around-the-clock opioids. Attention to bowel symptoms attendant to the use of opioids was also a key to improving patients' quality of life.

Beyond the management of physical symptoms, the modern hospice movement early on stressed attention to the needs of the whole person, including psychological, social, and spiritual suffering. A disease like cancer provides a scenario where death can be reasonably predicted within weeks or months. This knowledge of impending death creates the potential for added suffering as well as the opportunity to address this suffering. With most other diseases, when death will occur is far less certain, and the need to prepare for death is less evident.

The hospice model therefore developed as an interdisciplinary approach that was driven by the manifest needs of the patient and his or her family. If a patient's suffering was mostly spiritual, then chaplaincy was brought forward; if physical, medical professionals took the lead; and if social or psychological, the social workers and psychologists took charge. Often these issues could be addressed in a hierarchal fashion such that once physical concerns were addressed, psychosocial concerns and spiritual suffering could be attended to.

In spite of the fact that hospice care was initially developed in inpatient settings, there was also an understanding that continuity of care was needed in personal residences and other settings. If a patient's symptoms were managed well enough, they did not need to stay in an inpatient setting. Hospice care, especially in the United States but also in the United Kingdom, understood the need for hospice care in the home.

There was also the fundamental belief that preparation for death is part of the human experience, and people live as part of a family system—family being understood as those the patient is attached to, whether by blood, marriage, relationship, or proximity. Therefore patients and their families were always the unit of care. One of the best secrets of the success of hospice care is its ability to empower families to do more than they thought possible to provide care to the patient.

Six-Month Prognosis

Terminal illness has come to be defined as having a prognosis of 6 months or less. Hospice admission in many countries is tied to an estimated 6-month prognosis. This time period came about primarily because a significant number of cancer patients survive less than 6 months from the time their disease advances to a metastatic phase. This is the period when patients experience functional decline, and it corresponds to the period when there is the most opportunity to avoid unnecessary disease-modifying treatments.

Cancer patients with a limited prognosis and whose symptoms are managed can be cared for at home by family members taught to provide basic care. Hospice professionals effectively back them up with on-call services and short-term inpatient care. This is the basic model for hospice care in the United States that has developed over time.

HIV/AIDS

With the emergence of HIV/AIDS, there was considerable controversy over hospice's role. Initially, many U.K. and U.S. hospices were not in favor of caring for AIDS patients. However, it soon became apparent that AIDS—prior to the availability of highly active antiretroviral therapies (HAART)—was a relentless killer and that AIDS patients suffered many difficult physical, emotional, and spiritual symptoms that hospice care was designed to address. The U.S. National Hospice Organization (now the National Hospice and Palliative Care Organization, or NHPCO) advocated strongly that hospices had a duty to provide palliative care to people living with HIV/AIDS. Gradually, hospice programs became educated about managing the symptoms of HIV/AIDS, and by the late 1980s more than 5% of U.S. hospice patients had a diagnosis of HIV/AIDS.

Since the advent of HAART, thankfully the number of hospice patients with an HIV/AIDS diagnosis began to drop dramatically as the disease became more of a chronic illness. Still, however, there are a growing number of patients whose HAART therapies have failed or who are dying due to other factors. Hospices are once again admitting HIV/AIDS patients, usually for a short course of hospice care prior to death. Hospice AIDS deaths are now nowhere near the numbers seen in the 1980s and early 1990s, but it is still a concern.

Need for Hospice Care

Not everyone nearing death will need hospice or palliative care. Researchers have estimated that somewhere between 60% and 70% of all deaths will need palliative care in the time leading up to death (Connor, 1999; Stjernsward & Clarke, 2005). Those that will not use palliative care include the obvious sudden deaths from homicide, suicide, accidents, and injuries, but also non-HIV infectious disease deaths, patients who die from a sudden heart attack or stroke, and those who become acutely ill and die without a preceding period of disability or decline in functional ability.

Trajectories of Death

There are thought to be four main trajectories of death in the population (Lunney, Lynn, Foley, Lipson, & Guralnik, 2003). Sudden death from accidents, injuries, and homicide is the first trajectory, and except for bereavement support, this trajectory obviously does not need palliative care. The second trajectory can be thought of as the expected decline due to illness such as cancer, ALS, some HIV/AIDS, end-stage renal disease, and other progressive, fatal illnesses. Hospice care was initially designed for this population. The third trajectory covers those with solid organ failure, and the fourth trajectory covers those patients, usually very old, who are dying of the debility of old age, with or without a diagnosis of dementia. These patients also have problems that include infections, weight loss, Parkinson's, osteoporosis, and chronic long-standing conditions that may not be immediately life-threatening (such as prostate cancer in males).

The third and fourth groups have been particularly challenging for hospice and palliative care providers. There are clearly many needs for these patients that palliative care can respond to; however, it can be difficult to determine how long these patients will live. As with the HIV/AIDS population, hospices were initially reluctant to serve patients with these diagnoses. Again the NHPCO took the position that these patients have every right to hospice palliative care and began to develop guidance and educational materials to assist in decisions about admitting and caring for these patients.

Case Example

Take the example of a patient with congestive heart failure and chronic obstructive pulmonary disease. We will call the patient John. John was admitted to hospice in very poor condition. He was too weak and short of breath to get out of bed without assistance. His daughter, who lived across town, was able to provide some assistance, but she worked full time. John had lost considerable weight and his personal care was neglected. He was depressed and saw no purpose in continued life. After several months of hospice home care, including regular personal care and emotional support from the hospice team and regular visits from a volunteer, John improved to the point where he had gained weight, his shortness of breath was better managed with low-dose morphine, and his mood was improved.

After 9 months, the hospice team had to reconsider whether John's prognosis remained at 6 months or less. At 11 months, John was discharged from hospice with some ongoing contact. Three months later, after a call from John's daughter, John was readmitted in much worse condition. He died 2 days later. Such cases demonstrate the positive contributions to quality of life and survival made by hospice care (Connor, Pyenson, Fitch, & Spence, 2007), the ethical dilemmas faced at the end of life, and the difficulty of determining who will benefit from hospice care and when.

EFFORTS TO IMPROVE THE ACCURACY OF PROGNOSTICATION

Driving the issue of who should be receiving hospice care in the United States is a requirement that to be eligible, hospice patients must have a prognosis of 6 months or less, if the disease runs its normal course. Palliative care services have no explicit prognostic requirement but generally are aimed at patients with life-limiting illness. Since funding for hospice and palliative care is still scarce in most countries, patients with poorer prognoses tend to have priority to receive services, even when there is no explicit prognostic requirement.

As efforts to expand hospice care to noncancer patients in the United States grew more successful, there was an increasing need to improve the accuracy of prognostication primarily for patients with nonmalignant disease diagnoses. In 1995, NHPCO published the first set of *Medical Guidelines for Determining Prognosis in Selected Non-Cancer Diseases* (NHPCO, 1995). These guidelines attempted to give clinicians making prognostic judgments the kinds of questions they ought to address when making a decision about hospice referral, covering heart failure, chronic obstructive pulmonary disease, HIV/AIDS, kidney failure, liver failure, ALS, dementia, stroke, and coma.

While there was very limited research on prognosis with predictive validity for these diagnoses, the authors did the best they could with available evidence and expert opinion from top clinicians in these specialties. Still, the *Guidelines* proved not to be very accurate in determining who would die within 6 months. Prognostication remains more art than science, as it is practiced by physicians and others making decisions about hospice admission.

There has been criticism of the 6-month prognosis rule for hospice patients, particularly since the state of the science of prognostication is so limited. In Florida, the state licensing law for hospice allows for a prognosis of 12 months for hospice care; however, Medicare and Medicaid limit payment to patients with a 6-month prognosis. Most who work in hospice would agree that the 6-month prognostic requirement is a handicap. It can be a psychological barrier to a patient's willingness to be admitted and for physician referral to hospice. The dilemma is what to put in place of the 6-month rule. It would be better if we could use something like severity of illness or level of need for care. However, we lack the evidence to reliably establish such criteria for admission. We run the risk of substantially increasing the cost of hospice care if we disregard prognosis.

NHPCO initiated an effort to develop prognostic guidelines for selected cancers, particularly for hormonally mediated cancers such as breast and prostate; however, they were never published. The reluctance to further develop these guidelines stemmed, in part, from the fact that the Medicare fiscal intermediaries used the *Guidelines* to develop payment policies on hospice care. These local coverage decisions (formerly local medical review policies) turned the *Guidelines*, with some modification, into claim review policies, for which they were not intended. There is still debate over whether the *Guidelines* served to increase or limit access to hospice care in the United States. In the end, it appears that they have increased access for patients with noncancer diagnoses, as evidenced by the continued growth in admission of these patients. Steadily over the past decade, the proportion of hospice patients with cancer has decreased from 61.3% (2000) to 41.3% (2007), as shown in Figure 1. Cancer admissions do continue to grow, but the growth in noncancer admissions is far greater.

FIGURE 1. Decline in Proportion of U.S. Hospice Cancer Admissions 2000-2007

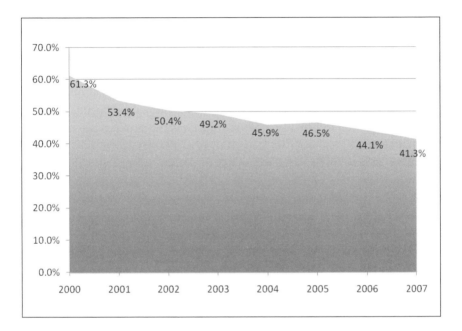

HOSPICE CARE FOR NONCANCER PATIENTS

Eventually the diagnostic mix of the hospice population is likely to reflect the chronically ill population dying in a given country. For the United States in 2006, 23% of all deaths were cancer deaths. If we assume that 70% of all deaths need palliative care, as previously proposed, and if we assume that 90% of cancer deaths need palliative care, then we could estimate that with full access, the percentage of hospice patients diagnosed with cancer would be approximately 30%—and that eventually, 70% of hospice patients will have noncancer diagnoses.

As noted in Figure 1, the current breakdown is about 40% cancer and 60% noncancer, so there will continue to be increased growth in the noncancer segment. To prepare for this growth, hospices need to align services with the needs of these patient populations. There will be increased need to develop new symptom management competencies. Patients with congestive heart failure have different needs than cancer patients. Hospice professionals need increased skill in managing congestive symptoms, for example, and understanding the risks associated with an arrhythmic death rather than death from gradual respiratory cessation.

In fact, it may be necessary to develop different care management and delivery models for the different trajectories of death experienced by noncancer patients. The solid-organ-failure patients may need care that is responsive to the problems associated with exacerbations of illness rather than a steadily increasing care delivery program as health declines and death approaches. For the frail elderly population, there may need to be more focus on practical assistance and personal care. Likewise, for patients with dementia, there is often a larger need to provide care that addresses the families' needs as long-term caregivers.

A host of new policy challenges has also come along with the growth in hospice care for noncancer patients. Due to Medicare hospice benefit regulations, hospices are required to discharge patients whose condition has improved to the point where they appear to have a prognosis greater than 6 months. The number of patients discharged from hospice for reasons other than death has been growing steadily along with the proportion of noncancer admissions (see Figure 2).

FIGURE 2. Growth in Live Discharges From U.S. Hospices 2002–2007

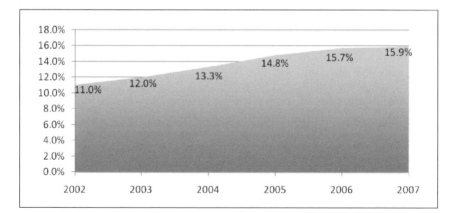

The dilemma, previously introduced, that patients improve with good palliative care to the point where they have to be discharged creates a difficult ethical challenge for hospices. Some have developed both pre- and posthospice follow-up programs to ameliorate this situation, providing varying degrees of contact and planned follow-up for patients and their families. The main objective of such programs is to monitor the patient's situation to ensure that hospice or palliative care can be reintroduced prior to death.

Some of the psychosocial concerns for noncancer patients also differ from those with cancer. Due to the more uncertain trajectory of noncancer diagnoses, there may be less urgency to deal with preparations for death. This can be misleading as the need for assistance with advance care planning may be even greater with a population more at risk for sudden death or cognitive decline.

Some less-enlightened regulators have questioned the need for hospice care for patients with dementing illnesses. Comments like "this patient cannot even communicate with you" indicate a lack of knowledge and sensitivity to the needs of patients and families facing this devastating illness. Not only do families of patients with dementia need large amounts of psychosocial support, there are tremendous needs for managing day-to-day care, respite needs, and very challenging treatment decisions that must be addressed.

One of the things palliative care workers have seen with the noncancer population is that, with good general management, there may be fewer extreme exacerbations of the underlying disease, resulting in fewer swings and gradual conversion to a more predictable decline in condition leading to death. This may make it easier to provide palliative care that comes closer to the cancer model.

FUTURE CONSIDERATIONS ABOUT CANCER AND NONCANCER CARE

As the hospice patient population mix has changed, there is also a need to reconsider how hospice care is delivered. No longer do we need a one-size-fits-all approach. The solid-organ-failure population will have periods of unchanged stability punctuated by extreme exacerbation of illness that will require intensive support. The frail elderly population will have a very slow downhill course, as will dementia patients who have to make key decisions about instituting or discontinuing treatments such as feeding tubes. Overall these patients will live longer with their illness than most cancer patients and will require more flexibility in how care is delivered.

It may be desirable to take more of a care-management approach to these patients. Such a model would call for thorough assessment, intensive care planning, and education at the start of care, followed by diminishing contact but with rapid response to any crisis situation that occurs.

The cancer trajectory is also changing. Due to advances in treatment, cancer is now becoming more of a chronic illness. The cancer death rate in the United States has actually declined, even though the absolute number of patients dying from cancer is increasing. This shift further underscores the need for hospice care to become more of a flexible model of care that is determined by the changing needs of the patients and families requiring service.

Hospice programs are also increasingly moving into the provision of general palliative care, usually in the form of providing consult services. This can be done in hospitals and nursing facilities, as well as the home or assisted living setting. Early hospice programs were primarily nurse led, while physicians played a fairly small role in overseeing care. Increasingly hospices are expanding physician staffing—not only to increase referrals, but also because physicians can generate enough revenues to pay for their services, especially by doing consults.

Community physicians are often more comfortable referring if they know the physician medical director and he or she has been certified in hospice and palliative medicine. The consult and care management approach may help hospices to reshape the model of hospice care that was originally developed for cancer patients. Those programs that adapt and build care delivery around the needs of patients and families and their different trajectories of illness will be more likely to thrive as our healthcare system undergoes dramatic changes. Given the aging of developed nations and the increasing need for balanced end-of-life care, it seems only right that hospice and palliative care will be a major part of the solution to the problems of our healthcare systems.

Stephen R. Connor, PhD, is the senior executive of the newly formed Worldwide Palliative Care Alliance (WPCA), an alliance of national hospice and palliative care organizations. He also serves as senior research and international consultant to the National Hospice and Palliative Care Organization (NHPCO) in Alexandria, Virginia, and is a part-time consultant to the Open Society Institute's International Palliative Care Initiative. Dr. Connor has worked continuously in the hospice/palliative care movement since 1976. In addition to being a hospice and association executive, he is a researcher and psychotherapist, licensed as a clinical psychologist in California and Kentucky. He has published over 50 peer-reviewed journal articles, reviews, and book chapters on issues related to palliative care for patients and their families and is the author of Hospice: Practice, Pitfalls, and Promise *(1998), and the just published book* Hospice and Palliative Care: The Essential Guide *(2009).*

References

Connor, S. (1995). Personal communication with Dr. Cicely Saunders, June 27, 1995, at International Work Group on Death, Dying, and Bereavement Conference in Oxford, England.

Connor, S. (1999). New initiatives transforming hospice care. *The Hospice Journal, 14*(3/4), 193–203.

Connor, S., Pyenson, B., Fitch, K., & Spence, C. (2007). Comparing hospice and non-hospice patient survival among patients who die within a 3-year window. *Journal of Pain and Symptom Management, 33*(3), 238–246.

Lunney, J. R., Lynn, J., Foley, D. J., Lipson, S., & Guralnik, J. M. (2003). Patterns of functional decline at the end of life. *JAMA, 289,* 2387–2392.

National Hospice and Palliative Care Organization. (1995). *Medical guidelines for determining prognosis in selected non-cancer diseases.* Alexandria, VA: Author.

Stjernsward, J., & Clarke, D. (2005). Palliative medicine—A global perspective. In D. Doyle, G. Hanks, N. Cherny, & K. Calman (Eds.), *Oxford textbook of palliative medicine.* Oxford, UK: Oxford University Press.

Difficult Choices: Making Decisions When Cure Is Not Possible

Stuart Farber

A life-threatening diagnosis creates a powerful new context in which a person and their family or community exist. The possibility of impending death becomes the context in which each day is lived when both patients and their families are confronted with the reality of mortality. They learn to cope not only with the uncertainty of the disease course, but also with the upheaval of personal worlds turned upside down. Projected futures are now unpredictable and often beyond their control (Farber, Egnew, Bertsch, Taylor, & Guldin, 2003). It is in this difficult context that patients with incurable cancer and their families must make complex medical decisions that have enormous consequences for all concerned: the patient, family members, and the medical team.

How does one make decisions that are congruent with the values and goals of a singular patient and family members in such a maelstrom of uncertainty and threat to life? Not easily, to be sure. The objective perspective of medicine presents a powerful way of viewing the world of the sick. From the perspective of the medical team as well as the patient and family, the concepts of diagnosis, prognosis, and treatment provide a way of understanding the experience of illness that is controllable and offers hope of actions that can prolong life. But the unique lived experience of the patient and family cannot be seen without going beyond the borders of the disease and its treatments. Yet asking a patient to articulate how her personal story might influence treatment is challenging. First, there are no places in the medical world for personal experience. Double-blind, randomized trials provide the gold standard of objective and reproducible information upon which sound medical decision making is based. The unique patient/family personal experience is suspect for its inability to be tested, quantified, or controlled. Second, for the patient and family living with the losses and limitations of advancing illness, complex treatments and the daily struggle to survive take precedence over reflecting on the quality of life one wants to live (Farber et al., 2003).

Take, for example, Jessie, a 55-year-old woman with advanced lung cancer who is nearing the end of her life when she develops the common complication of pneumonia. The physician leads the treatment discussion from the medical perspective, considering diagnosis, prognosis, and treatment, as well as from an innate belief in the value of taking action to modify disease, especially to prevent death (Weissman, 2004). The physician's logic pulls everyone in its wake:

1. *Diagnosis*: Bacterial infection of the lung.
2. *Prognosis*: Death likely without treatment; recovery possible with treatment.
3. *Treatment*: Antibiotic is simple, noninvasive, and highly effective; nontreatment is abandonment and physical suffering.
4. *Conclusion*: Antibiotic treatment of pneumonia is doing something to promote life; nontreatment is doing nothing, leading to death and suffering.

The physician leads from the medical perspective without considering the patient or family lived experience. Pausing to wonder "Is this a good day for Jessie to die?" is taboo by the logic of the discussion. To ask such a question would require extraordinary courage of Jessie and her family. The possibility of pneumonia being medically managed to prevent suffering and allowing a peaceful death is an unknown option, even though preventing death at this moment is only delaying the next life-threatening crisis that will surface in the near future. The central question, "Is there more quality life to live?" from the singular perspective of Jessie and her family has not been asked. The answer is essential for the physician, Jessie, and the family to cocreate a treatment plan that respects the values and goals of Jessie and her family while acknowledging the medical reality (Farber et al., 2003).

This chapter explores how a more complex and creative process of decision making can emerge from the present medically dominated approach. While acknowledging the importance of medicine's role and the marvel of modern technology in cancer treatment, I simultaneously explore the value of moving beyond medicine's world to incorporate the rich tapestry of personal human experience. In the intricate process of living the end of life, there are many experts who need to work together. The medical team is expert at treating serious illness, and patients and families are experts in knowing what gives their lives meaning and value. Bringing together each party's expertise will cocreate a future with the deepest meaning and value (Farber, Egnew, & Farber, 2004).

UNDERSTANDING CANCER AND ITS TREATMENTS

The explosion of knowledge about cancer over the past 30 years is staggering and continues to accelerate. Genomics (the study of the entire genetic code of a cell) and molecular genetics (the study of specific genes) are providing a deeper understanding of what causes cancer and generating new, more targeted treatments.

Patients and families have differing attitudes on how much they wish to know about the medical aspects of their diagnosis. Some want to know as much as their physician. Others want broad concepts but are not interested in details. For physicians, a central task under the concept of informed consent is sharing with a patient the details of the cancer and its treatments, creating a potential conflict. An important process that is often not addressed by physicians is negotiating just how much information a patient or family desires and how this information is best communicated. This negotiation is a critical first step.

USING NARRATIVE TO COCREATE A MEDICAL PLAN

A fundamental challenge facing a patient, family members, and the medical team is how to relate to each other so that medical decisions are made collaboratively in a way that meaningfully includes patient/family values and goals. This is inherently difficult due to the life-and-death nature of the situation and the power imbalance among the patient, family, and medical team. The patient and family are often novices in the world of illness. Each decision has enormous consequences that are difficult to appreciate in advance. The patient and family experience a steep learning curve as every major decision deepens their understanding. This experiential learning results in the patient and family constantly changing and growing through their experience (Farber et al., 2003).

Agreeing to a new round of chemotherapy takes on a drastically different meaning after completing the first cycle. Physicians and other healthcare professionals have broad experience in end-of-life care and maintain a relatively stable understanding of the treatment experience. After caring for 200 patients with pancreatic cancer, caring for the 201st patient is not going to significantly change the perspective of an experienced physician. Adding to this imbalance is the difficulty for everyone—including physicians—of facing mortality (Callahan, 1994). It is little wonder then that more than two thirds of Americans die in hospitals and nursing homes, often receiving life-prolonging care up to the last moments of life. Few physicians recognize when a patient is dying, and fewer patients and families are aware that they are living the end of their lives. Doing things to stay alive takes precedence over living a quality life until death comes (Field & Cassel, 1997; Kaufman, 2005).

In this cauldron of disease, loss, pain, hope, fear, and treatments, how do the physician, the patient, and the family shift the focus from doing things to stay alive to doing things to live a life of value and meaning? First, it should be recognized that few complex life decisions are based on only rational, linear reasoning. Very few people pick their spouse using criteria defined on an Excel spreadsheet. Most of us use narrative (our story) to make meaning out of our lives and to guide our decisions. Our narratives are a multilayered way to make sense out of conflicting facts, emotions, hopes, and fears that we experience in life (Cassell, 1991; Kaufman, 1986). Transparent and shared patient, family, and physician stories allow for balancing medical decisions on both facts and patient/family values (Farber et al., 2004).

Narrative medicine is a term coined in the early 1990s to describe the concept of using the illness stories "told" by patients and carefully "heard" by physicians to guide medical care (Charon, 2001). I propose that it is the responsibility of everyone involved in a patient's care to explore, clarify, and share narratives. By doing so, a common story is created that allows shared values to cocreate the future of the patient, family, and medical team. It is critical that physicians and the medical team find out from the patient and family members what they already know, what they want to know, and what they need to know beyond the medical facts (Farber et al., 2004; Sackett, Strauss, Richardson, Rosenberg, & Haynes, 2000).

Let me share a practical example. John, a rancher from Montana, came to a regional referral center to receive a nonrelated-donor bone marrow transplant for a form of leukemia. He and his family expected either a miraculous cure or death from complications of the transplant. Neither occurred. The transplant was "successful" in that the new bone marrow engrafted (took), but simultaneously it severely attacked John's body (skin and digestive system) as foreign (graft versus host disease, GVHD). Despite all attempts to suppress the GVHD, John continued to have severe rashes, bloody diarrhea, and abdominal pain. His medical team described his condition as "incurable" but "controllable" and noted that he "might" get better. John was told he needed even stronger immunosuppressive drugs and intravenous feeding or he would die. He consented, hoping he would get "better." Despite all treatments, 2 months later he was still in the hospital having survived two ICU stays for severe infections induced by his immunosuppressive drugs. While these drugs improved his GVHD, they also reduced his immune system to the point where normal bacteria caused life-threatening infections.

At this point a palliative care consult was requested, which facilitated the sharing of narratives. The medical team told their story: It was still possible to try experimental drugs to improve John's situation and keep him alive longer. He had a 25% chance of improving with the new drug regimen. John then stated clearly his goals for medical treatment: He wanted to get enough better to return to his ranch in Montana, to be with his family, and to ride his horse on his property. Palliative care then asked the medical team to comment on whether the treatments they were offering could meet John's goals. The medical team stated clearly that John's goals were unobtainable with his present treatment plan. The drugs were experimental and could be provided only in the hospital. While these drugs might prolong his life, eventually he would die in the hospital from his GVHD. His death might be months from now, but they had never seen anyone as sick as John return home.

At the conclusion of this meeting, John stated with conviction that his goal remained to return to his ranch. If he was going to die, he wanted it to be in his own home surrounded by all that was important to him. The sharing of narratives allowed John to decide how medical treatments could support him to live a quality life until he died. He and his family chose to go home with hospice support. Without the sharing of narratives, John most certainly would have died in the hospital. When John's medical team contained his story within the linear world of statistics and test results, they could not grasp the more complex issues that allowed them to understand what was most important to John.

THE LIMITS OF QUANTITATIVE METHODS IN CLINICAL DECISION MAKING

Physicians use objective, quantitative information as the fulcrum point for making medical decisions. What is rarely made clear in discussions with patients are the limitations of this approach. I will first discuss some important implications of using statistical probability to guide individual decisions, and then explore the use of statistics and objective tests in deciding treatments of uncertain benefit.

Statistical methods are used to describe the probability of what will happen within a group. The larger the group, the more powerful statistics are at predicting outcomes. In terms of medical care, for example, statistics are used to describe the results of large studies on different treatments for cancer. The most respected studies are double-blind, randomized controlled trials. In such studies the experimental treatment is often compared to the commonly accepted best current treatment. No one knows who is getting what treatment, so bias is reduced. The information gained from such trials is important in determining which new treatments are best for a particular cancer. The challenge comes in interpreting what these statistical results mean for a singular patient. In fact, applying statistics to an individual case is really a misapplication of statistical methods. The standard deviation (variation) in the individual case is unpredictable.

In practical terms, a patient will not be 70% dead or 30% alive after 5 years. They will either be 100% alive or 100% dead. Thus from the patient's and physician's perspective, the future is unpredictable. You will know the outcome only after you have received the treatment. This precept holds even when the likelihood of a positive outcome is very high. Say 99% of people taking the antibiotic amoxicillin for pneumonia improve, and less than 0.01% have a life-threatening complication. If you have a life-threatening complication, it is 100% of your experience (Feinstein, 1994). The same caution required by the Securities and Exchange Commission when investing in the stock market applies to using statistics when making medical decisions: "Past performance is no guarantee of future results."

The use of statistics and objective tests in deciding whether to take chemotherapy in far-advanced cancer is a particularly complex process. Again statistics are used to describe the benefits. Say a patient has advanced pancreatic cancer. The physician can say 27% of patients respond to the agent gemcitabine. In those patients who received the drug versus those patients who received the former standard treatment of 5-fluorouracil (5-FU), response may be defined as either decrease in tumor size on imaging (11% respond), or improvement in functional status, that is, less pain, less weight loss, better performance status (27% respond). As a patient is making her decision, she needs to consider several factors. The first is the effect on survival. In this case, the median survival with gemcitabine was 5.65 months, compared with 4.41

months with 5-FU (Burris et al., 1997). Thus the patient will want to weigh the potential of a relatively short increase in her life versus the time spent receiving chemotherapy and its potential side effects. Second, as a singular patient she doesn't have a 27% chance of benefit. If she responds to gemcitabine, she will have a 100% outcome of benefit (responder). If she doesn't respond, she will have a 100% outcome of no benefit (nonresponder). Before taking the drug, there is no way to tell whether she is a responder or a nonresponder. Trying the drug is the only way to find out.

Here is a specific example. Saul had a far-advanced gastrointestinal-stromal-tumor (GIST). He enrolled in a Phase III investigational study of a new chemotherapy. He received the first round of treatments and became severely ill with nausea, vomiting, and diarrhea. Saul was hospitalized on multiple occasions for dehydration, weakness, weight loss, and pain. As he recovered from his initial round of treatment, he had imaging to measure the tumor's response. The radiologist and oncologist thought the tumor had shrunk 10%–15% in some areas and grown significantly in others. Saul talked with the oncologist, who said he wasn't sure if the new agent was helping but offered a second round of treatment. After careful reflection and discussion with a palliative care clinician, Saul understood that he was a nonresponder and that the chemo was making his life miserable. In fact, the experimental treatment was more likely shortening his life and certainly diminishing the quality of his life. He opted out of the study. Saul's oncologist's focus on "objective information" blinded him to the fact that no CT scan can measure the amount of suffering experienced by Saul and his family or, as attributed to Albert Einstein, "Not everything that can be counted counts, and not everything that counts can be counted."

THE CHALLENGE OF PARADOX

Choosing among unknowns is daunting. We live constantly in paradox. Webster's defines paradox as "a statement that is seemingly contradictory or opposed to common sense and yet is perhaps true." Let's explore three paradoxes that influence decision making for everyone living with advanced cancer: patient, family, physician, and health care team.

- We are simultaneously living and dying.
- We are simultaneously certain and uncertain about our future.
- We are simultaneously autonomous individuals and interdependent members of a community.

Paradox means holding two seemingly incompatible truths, which may create dissonance and tension. Resolving paradox into one truth reduces or eliminates this tension. Desiring to resolve paradox is a strong human trait that is deeply engrained in our culture. Living in paradox requires accepting dissonance, no easy task for most of us (Palmer, 1998). Let us examine paradox and explore its effects on decision making.

WE ARE SIMULTANEOUSLY LIVING AND DYING

Physicians focus on living. Every effort to prolong life is the central enterprise of medical practice. Despite this effort, patients die and physicians must accommodate. Most often, physicians handle the life/death paradox by resolving it into two parts. As long as there are medical treatments that can prolong life without inordinate suffering, then from the doctor's perspective a patient is "living." Once there are no medical treatments that can reasonably prolong the patient's life without inordinate suffering, then the patient is "dying" (Kaufman, 2005).

The clinical consequences of this approach are powerful. First, it delays any meaningful discussion of death until very late in the trajectory of illness, usually days or even hours before death. Second, it is difficult for the physician to know when a patient is actually dying. Instead of measuring mortality by the physiologic decline of advancing disease, mortality is measured by the effectiveness of medical treatments from the objectified culture of medicine (Kaufman, 2005). Jessie with lung cancer and pneumonia, John with severe GVHD, and Saul with GIST were all dying, yet none of their physicians ever openly recognized or discussed this obvious fact. Why not? Because there were more treatments to potentially extend life that put each of these patients in the "living" category. Researchers, including the Dartmouth Institute for Health Policy and Clinical Practice, are now challenging the assumption that more medical care is better. Analyzing Medicare data for chronically ill patients in the last two years of life, these researchers have concluded that "more" increases cost without improving quality or outcomes (Connor, Pyenson, Fitch, Spence, & Iwasaki, 2007; Wennberg, Fisher, Goodman, & Skinner, 2008).

If the physician has trouble accommodating the fact a patient is dying, how are the patient and family members supposed to make this recognition independently? In fact, both Saul and John lived deeply fulfilling lives once they transitioned their medical care toward goals consistent with their narratives. Both they and their families stated that the last days were deeply rich and meaningful in a way that could not have occurred without acknowledging mortality as part of life.

We Are Simultaneously Certain and Uncertain About Our Future

Physicians understand that uncertainty exists but view it as an uncomfortable reality that should be minimized. The use of statistics and probabilities are powerful, objective ways to manage uncertainty. Physicians focus on what they know and can control as a way to create certainty in an uncertain situation. In the example of the patient with advanced pancreatic cancer on gemcitibine, the likelihood of death in the next 6–12 months is greater than 95%. Yet no one (patient, physician, or family) has any idea of exactly how or when death will occur. The physician is both certain death will occur and uncertain as to when or how it will happen. By focusing on what the physician does know and can treat, an aura of certainty envelops an inherently uncertain situation and provides the illusion that living is being supported and death is being prevented (Hall, 2002; West & West, 2002).

From the perspective of the ill person and his or her family, uncertainty is a source of both anxiety and hope. "While more than 95% of patients with advanced pancreatic cancer will be dead within a year, perhaps I will be one of those who survive." In fact, this will be true for a few. Thus the ill person lives with "uncertain certainty." The most certain information that the patient possesses is knowing her or his values and goals. What defines quality of life, meaning, and purpose usually is quite clear to the ill person and family. John with GVHD was absolutely certain he wanted to go back to his ranch. Saul with GIST was also certain he wanted to discontinue his chemotherapy based on his definition of quality of life. Unfortunately, John's physician didn't gain a meaningful understanding of the patient/family narrative until a palliative care consult extremely late in John's disease course. Saul's oncologist never did.

We Are Simultaneously Autonomous Individuals and Interdependent Members of a Community

The concept of autonomy is embedded in our general culture and particularly in medicine. The American ideal of self-reliance and the right of an individual to decide what she or he will do in every aspect of life is codified in our laws. Medical ethics has raised the value of autonomy to such a high level, it has become a trump card that generally negates other competing values such as beneficence, nonmalfeasance, and justice. The reality is no one who is seriously ill lives an autonomous life. Patients live in a dynamic community where each member's decisions impact every other member.

This high value on autonomy has dramatic effects on care at the end of life. One of the most powerful examples is determining care at the moment of death. For clinicians, such discussions are termed "determining code status." A common approach is to ask Saul with his far-advanced GIST what he wants done if he stops breathing or his heart stops. Does he want to be allowed to die, or does he want to be resuscitated? Given Saul's advanced illness, if resuscitation is provided, he will never leave the hospital alive. Rather than supporting his life, it will prolong his dying and assure he dies isolated from his family (in the intensive care unit) while receiving highly technical care (Kaufman, 2005). So why do physicians offer a costly treatment that has no measurable benefit and almost certainly will cause suffering and harm? Based on the principles of beneficence, nonmalfeasance, and justice, resuscitation should not be offered, but autonomy demands that Saul makes the final choice, albeit with limited knowledge.

There is excellent documentation on the powerful effects providing such treatments has on physicians and medical students (Jackson et al., 2005; Kearney, Weininger, & Vaschon, 2009; Rhodes-Kropf et al., 2005). Saul's choice not only affects him, but everyone else involved. Families spend the final hours and days in hospital intensive care units being asked to make further decisions about more invasive care or, more difficult, withdrawing care (Kaufman, 2005). This scenario is occurring repeatedly in U.S. hospitals with no measurable benefit in quality of life for anyone. It is as if the "final rights" of passage that once were in the hands of priests, rabbis, and ministers are now in the hands of high-tech medicine.

Another important aspect is that no one generally explores *why* a patient chooses to be resuscitated. In Saul's case, he had an 8-month-pregnant granddaughter who was very dear to him. She had told her grandfather that it was important to her for Saul to see and bless his great-grandchild. From Saul's perspective, resuscitation may allow him to achieve this goal. When his physician gave him a choice, Saul did not know that that he was being offered a treatment that had no measurable benefit and would cause more suffering.

LIVING IN PARADOX BY "EXPECTING THE BEST WHILE PREPARING FOR EVERYTHING"

So how can clinicians and patients and their families find a way to live in the paradoxes of incurable cancer? There is no simple answer, but here is a phrase I use repeatedly in my work to assist in moving toward living in the paradox. Imagine you are speaking to Saul, John, or Jessie: "We are always expecting the best, and at the same time preparing for everything that can happen, including the worst. We need to make sure we understand what you and your family define as the best in the difficult situation that we are all facing. We also need to explore what you define as the worst." By using such language, palliative care physicians facilitate several goals simultaneously.

First, we reinforce that the "best," however defined by the patient and family, is still potentially obtainable. Second, we allow the patient and family to hold onto their hope while simultaneously creating back-up plans for less desirable outcomes. The patient and family don't have to choose between getting better (living) and getting worse (dying). They can prepare for both outcomes at the same time. Third, we are asking the patient and family to define the "best" and "worst" outcomes from their perspectives. As we explore the best and worst, we help them clarify their values and goals. The knowledge gained will assist in cocreating a future that is built upon the foundation of these patient and family values and goals. Often there will be conflicting narratives among the patient, family, and medical team. However, airing these differences enables us to focus on the patient- and family-defined goals and has the potential to radically alter decision making at the end of life. It ensures that medical care provided is respectful of the patient/family narrative (Farber et al., 2004; Tulsky, 2005).

While the best for a few patients is to live to their biologic maximum, for many patients living a comfortable and meaningful life is most important. Certainly this was the case for both Saul and John. Each patient and family will have a singular set of definitions for what is meaningful, and it is central to the conversation to assist them in sharing their illness narrative and the best ending from their perspective. Likewise the worst for a few patients will be death in any form, but for the majority, a painful, prolonged, technologic death filled with suffering is what is feared most (Field & Cassel, 1997; Kaufman, 2005). This is the scenario that was being lived by Saul and John until a transition to care more respectful of their narratives occurred. Each transition occurred because a clinician had the time and skill to help explore their narratives and clarify goals and values.

DEVELOPMENTAL OPPORTUNITIES WHILE LIVING WITH CANCER

Saul, John, and their families all shared that the last weeks of life were some of the richest and most meaningful they had ever experienced. Research and personal narrative in end-of-life care confirm that the opportunities for personal growth and development are profound and potentially transformative (Byock, 1997; Chochinov, 2002; McPhee & Markowitz, 2001). There is something about accepting mortality that creates an intensity and authenticity of living that no other time in the life cycle can create. In Thornton Wilder's play *Our Town*, Emily asks the stage manager, "Do any human beings ever realize life while they live it—every, every minute?" The manager replies, "No, saints and poets maybe—they do some" (Wilder, 1938). I would add, "And so do many patients and families living the end of life." One of the greatest morbidities of our present death-denying system is that patients and families are so extremely ill when they recognize they are at the end of life, they have neither the time nor the energy to take advantage of this time that many cultures call sacred.

Stuart Farber, MD, has devoted his career to issues in end-of-life care. He is board certified in family medicine, hospice, and palliative medicine. He is a Project on Death in America scholar; founder and director of the University of Washington Medical Center's Palliative Care Consult Service; a published researcher; and an associate professor in the Department of Family Medicine at the University of Washington School of Medicine. After 17 years of practicing family medicine in an urban community, Dr. Farber returned to academic medicine to pursue research and education in end-of-life care. His projects include qualitative research from the clinician, patient, and family perspectives; development of courses for health science students in hospice, spirituality, and chronic advanced illness; and systems approaches to improving pain management and decision making for patients with life-threatening illnesses. He is a founding member and past chairperson of the Washington State End-of-Life Consensus Coalition, a broad-based community organization to promote discussion and improvement in end-of-life care for all citizens in the state.

REFERENCES

Burriss, H. A., Moore, M. J., Anderson, J., Green, M. R., Rothenberg, M. L., Modiano, M. R., et al. (1997). Improvement in survival and clinical benefit with gemcitabine as first-line therapy for patients with advanced pancreatic cancer: A randomized trial. *Journal of Clinical Oncology, 15,* 2403–2413.

Byock, I. (1997). *Dying well.* New York: Riverhead Books.

Callahan, D. (1994). *The troubled dream of life: In search of a peaceful death.* New York: Touchstone Books/Simon and Schuster.

Cassell, E. (1991). *The nature of suffering and the goals of medicine.* Oxford, England: Oxford University Press.

Charon, R. (2001). Narrative medicine: A model for empathy, reflection, profession, and trust. *JAMA, 286,* 1897–1902.

Chochinov, H. M. (2002). Dignity-conserving care—A new model for palliative care: Helping the patient feel valued. *JAMA, 287,* 2253–2259.

Connor, S. R., Pyenson, B., Fitch, K., Spence, C., & Iwasaki, K. (2007). Comparing hospice and nonhospice patient survival among patients who die within a three year window. *Journal of Pain and Symptom Management, 33,* 238–246.

Farber, S., Egnew, T. R., Bertsch, J., Taylor, T. R., & Guldin, G. (2003). Issues in end-of-life care: Patient, caregiver, and clinician perceptions. *Journal of Palliative Medicine, 6,* 19–31.

Farber, S., Egnew, T. R., & Farber, A. (2004). What is a respectful death? In J. Borzoff & P. Silverman (Eds.), *Living with dying* (Part II, ch. 5). New York: Columbia University Press.

Feinstein, A. R. (1994). Clinical judgment revisited: The distraction of quantitative models. *Annals of Internal Medicine, 120,* 799–805.

Field, M., & Cassel, C. (1997). *Approaching death.* Washington, DC: Institute of Medicine.

Hall, K. H. (2002). Reviewing intuitive decision-making and uncertainty: The implications for medical education. *Medical Education, 36,* 216–224.

Jackson, V. A., Sullivan, A. M., Gadmer, N. M., Seltzer, D., Mitchell, A. M., Lakoma, M. D., et al. (2005). "It was haunting …": Physician's descriptions of emotionally powerful patient deaths. *Academic Medicine, 80,* 648–656.

Kaufman, S. R. (1986). *The ageless self.* Madison, WI: University of Wisconsin Press.

Kaufman, S. R. (2005). *And a time to die: How American hospitals shape the end of life.* Madison, WI: University of Wisconsin Press.

Kearney, M. K., Weininger, R. B., & Vaschon, M. L. S. (2009). Self-care of physicians caring for patients at the end of life: "Being connected … a key to my survival." *JAMA, 301,* 1155–1164.

McPhee, S. J., & Markowitz, A. J. (2001). Psychological considerations, growth and transcendence at the end of life: The art of the possible. *JAMA, 286,* 3002.

Palmer P. J. (1998). *The courage to teach* (ch. 3). San Francisco: Jossey-Bass.

Rhodes-Kropf, J., Carmody, S. S., Seltzer, D., Redenbaugh, E., Gadmer, N., Block, S. D., et al. (2005). "This is just too awful; I just can't believe I experienced that …": Medical students' reactions to their "most memorable" patient death. *Academic Medicine, 80,* 634–640.

Sackett, D. L., Strauss, S. E., Richardson, W. S., Rosenberg, W., & Haynes, R. B. (2000). *Evidence based medicine.* Edinburgh: Churchill Livingstone.

Tulsky, J. A. (2005). Beyond advance directives: Importance of communication skills at the end of life. *JAMA, 294,* 359–365.

Weissman, D. E. (2004). Decision making at a time of crisis near the end of life. *JAMA, 292,* 1738–1743.

Wennberg, J. E., Fisher, E. S., Goodman, D. C., & Skinner, J. S. (2008). Tracking the care of patients with severe chronic illness, executive summary. In *The Dartmouth atlas of health care 2008.* Dartmouth, NH: Dartmouth Institute for Health Care Policy and Clinical Practice.

West, A. F., & West, R. R. (2002). Clinical decision-making: Coping with uncertainty. *Post Graduate Medicine, 78,* 319–321.

Wilder, T. (1938). *Our town: Acting edition.* New York: Coward-McCann Inc. in cooperation with Samuel French Inc.

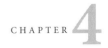

After the Battle, Journeys with Cancer: Changing Metaphors of Illness

Neil Small

IN PRAISE OF SUSAN SONTAG

In 1978, Susan Sontag published a short book, *Illness as Metaphor*, in which she argued that "the most truthful way of regarding illness—and the healthiest way of being ill—is one most purified, most resistant to metaphoric thinking" (Sontag, 1991, p. 3).[1] There are some metaphors, she argued, that "we might well try to abstain from or to retire" (p. 91). Cancer (and before it, tuberculosis) have been "spectacularly and similarly encumbered by the trappings of metaphor" (p. 5), and these encumbrances have cost lives. Cancer, she argued, "is just a disease" (p. 100).

The spur to writing *Illness as Metaphor* was her own diagnosis and treatment for cancer. "When I became a cancer patient," she writes, "what particularly enraged me—and distracted me from my own terror and despair at my doctors' gloomy prognosis—was seeing how much the very reputation of this illness added to the suffering of those who had it" (Sontag, 1991, p. 97).

Illness as Metaphor still constitutes such a significant intervention in the way we understand illness that any consideration of metaphor in cancer, and in other life-limiting illness, requires an engagement with, and development of, Sontag's work.

The case Sontag presents builds on a historical critique that there have been a series of master illnesses, most recently tuberculosis (TB) and then cancer, and these illnesses accumulate controlling metaphors. Cancer's is drawn from the language of warfare, which renders cancer mortifying and it becomes both shaming and silencing. Shaming means people do not seek help early enough,

---

1 All page numbers in *Illness as Metaphor* and *AIDS and Its Metaphors* refer to an edition published by Penguin Books in 1991 that combines both books into one volume.

while silencing means that one person with cancer cannot be informed by the experience of another. Sontag wanted people not to delay going to the doctor and to feel able to change their doctors and to question the treatment they were given. She wanted to encourage people to be less fearful of cancer treatments, specifically chemotherapy, and to be able to resist "useless remedies" such as "diets and psychotherapy." These aims locate *Illness as Metaphor* as an active intervention in health politics. But it was also a cultural intervention. Its approach was intertextual. That is, it developed its argument at the interface of a reading of literature and of Sontag's own illness narrative. It is this coming together of the personal and the poetic that gives the book much of its power to persuade.

Eleven years later, Sontag presented *AIDS and Its Metaphors*. Much had changed. She was then cured of her cancer and she had identified a number of changes in the social position of cancer. In these intervening years, she identified a reduction in the stigma associated with getting cancer: Cancer was talked about more; diagnoses were now shared (at least in the United States); there was a greater public profile with details of individuals' experiences of cancer now in the public domain. By 1989, she was also able to argue that cancer had lost its position as the master illness. It was no longer the most feared disease. That status, she believed, had transferred to AIDS.

I propose to consider the salience of Sontag's position in 2009, 31 years after *Illness as Metaphor* and 20 years after *AIDS and Its Metaphors*. The key elements of the case she was making were that there are master illnesses that change over time; that there are controlling metaphors associated with these illnesses; that at the time she was writing, cancer was the master illness and the controlling metaphor was a military one. Further, she argued that some metaphors are mortifying. That is, they make the experience of the illness worse, and that the best way to be ill is a way free of metaphorical interpretation. I will take each of these elements and reflect on Sontag's justification for making them in 1978 and 1989 and the extent to which they are valuable descriptors of the cancer experience today.

Sontag had too narrow a definition of metaphor, and when she was writing there were other metaphors that people drew on. She also overstated her case that "silence and shame *invariably* characterize the cancer experience" (Clow, 2001, p. 294). Today, there are not such controlling metaphors due to a continuing shift toward a proliferation of languages of signification—a shift captured in the idea of a move from modernity to postmodernity. We have not disposed of metaphors. Rather, we live surrounded by multiple metaphors. Our relationship with them is not one of struggling against domination but of choosing between options.

MASTER ILLNESSES

Patterson calls Sontag's "master illness" a "dread disease" (Patterson, 1987). Different illnesses have occupied the role of master illness: leprosy, syphilis, cholera, TB, cancer. These illnesses have shared features: they are mysterious, transformative as the body becomes something alienating, and fatal. But a disease only achieves master status through the interchange between the disease and the prevailing society. The master disease represents "the worm in the bud." It captures our deepest dread not just because of the corruption and decay it visits on the body, but the hubris it reveals in society. In this way, industrialization brought about the fear of enforced proximity and the dread of tuberculosis. Modernity assumed the harmony of reason and progress. Its offspring was science, whose favored son was medicine. Given time, growth (of knowledge and capacity) would solve all problems. Cancer has exactly the characteristics to deflate this expectation. Growth (of cells) was out of control and destructive. We see then the struggle, or war, between modernist optimism with its faith in reason and science and elusive, mysterious, transformative cancer.

But there have been changes in the manifestations of cancer: how many live with it and how long they are alive. For many people, cancer will be considered a chronic, controllable condition. There are also changes in the way that we engage with science. While there has long been an assumption that science will continue to accrue knowledge about cancer, and while in recent years there has been a step change in how much we know about causes and about the various stages it takes as it progresses in and through the cells of the body, there are many uncertainties about key processes. We can see how it is possible to know much about what happens in any cellular process but not why it happens in a specific case or what precisely starts the process. We are now able to have a more nuanced appreciation of the limits of reason and the power of science. Consequently, we are a little better at distinguishing between scientific optimism and therapeutic caution. This allows us to consider metaphors of cancer that are neither militaristic nor punitive. Cancer can be thought of as different things at the same time.

This sense of coexisting possibilities and different interpretations is characteristic of postmodernism. This involves embracing curious unknowing, "getting people to no longer know what to do so that things might be done differently" (Lather, 2007, p. 152). This is an epistemology that privileges doubt and renounces universality but it contains features that resonate with its own dread disease, its new master illness. There is an imperative in uncertain times to shape one's own narrative, to exercise choice. Not being able to choose becomes transformative of the self, alienating and mysterious. Dementia is quintessentially identified with a loss of this autonomous self. As such, it resonates with a particular spirit of the time and achieves master status via a reciprocal interchange between the manifestations of the disease and the prevailing characteristic of society.

Understanding Metaphor[2]

We have always used metaphor, although what we understand it to be is contested. Sontag recognized that "one cannot think without metaphors…. As, of course, all thinking is interpretation" (Sontag, 1991, p. 91). But her focus is an understanding of metaphor as defined by Aristotle in *Poetics*. Metaphor is, "giving a thing a name that belongs to something else," a rhetorical device (Sontag, 1991, p. 91). But others have seen metaphor as broader, as integral to the system of language as "human thought processes are largely metaphorical…. The human conceptual system is metaphorically saturated and defined" (Lakoff & Johnson, 1980, p. 6). Ricoeur (1986) goes beyond metaphor as rhetorical, semantic, or conceptual and argues that metaphor is something we live through—that it resides in our ontology. The very way knowledge is produced is steeped in metaphor.

If metaphor is rhetorical and we recognize that some metaphors have unintended mortifying effects, we can either keep using them, choose less damaging metaphors, or seek to eliminate metaphor from illness altogether. If it is integral to language, it is diffused across our general approach to illness and may not even be apparent to us. If it is ontological, then we need to consider if we can even conceive of some things without metaphor. An example can be drawn from Michel Foucault's influential work on the different ways medicine

---

2 This section was developed while reading Jackie Stacey's book, *Teratologies* (1997). Stacey was diagnosed with cancer in 1991 and her book combines the autobiographical with a cultural study of the way cancer is perceived, experienced, and theorized. This is a combination reminiscent of Sontag's work with which it shares an eloquence and power but from which it differs in that Stacey remains committed to analyzing the cancer narrative as contrasted with Sontag's modernist stance against interpretation.

has been imagined. He identifies organizing metaphors of space and vision that encapsulate the parameters of the possible and shape the focus of what medicine can "see."

Foucault, in his archaeology of medicine (1973), identifies a shift from a medicine of classification, essentially constructed around a spatial metaphor, to a clinico-anatomical medicine where the defining metaphor is one of vision. It was a process in which "a grammar of signs... replaced a botany of symptoms" (p. xviii). In classificatory medicine the patient and the disease are considered to be separate. For example, "The same spasmodic malady...may move around the body causing dyspepsia in the lower abdomen, palpitations in the chest and epileptic convulsions in the head" (p. 14). In contrast, in clinico-anatomical medicine the disease is isolated and divided into closed regions of the body. "This new structure is indicated in the change in the doctor's question from 'what's the matter with you?' to 'where does it hurt?'" (Stacey, 1997, p. 54).

If metaphor is more than rhetorical, we cannot dispense with it. All illnesses are inseparable from the meanings ascribed to them within their specific cultural location (Stacey, 1997; DiGiacomo, 1992) and all these ascribed meanings are imbued with the metaphorical—even Western biomedicine. But perhaps we can identify different levels of metaphor, some that are rhetorical and some that organize our perceptions of the possible.

VARIETY OF METAPHOR:
BEFORE AND CONTEMPORANEOUS WITH SONTAG

There was indeed evidence for conspiracies of silence and a prevalence of euphemisms before and at the time Susan Sontag was writing. Physicians would either not tell people of the diagnosis or dissemble in a way that allowed patients and families to shun or avoid the diagnosis while obituaries and death notices talked of "lingering illnesses." But, as Clow has argued, this was not the full picture. There was coverage of cancer in newspapers, magazines, and local radio. People with cancer consulted friends, neighbors, medical specialists, alternative healers, and informal networks (Clow, 2001, p. 301). There were also book-length personal accounts of illness, what Hawkins called "pathographies" (Hawkins, 1993, pp. 3–5). By the time *Illness as Metaphor* was published, Hawkins had identified a change in the prevailing stance in these. Those written in the immediate post-Second World War years celebrated the possibilities of modern medicine. Those written later, but still before Sontag, were mistrustful of the medical establishment. This is supportive of the shift from modernism described above. Sontag was out of step with the prevailing approach, perhaps not surprising given her source material was her own experiences and her library.

Further, an assumption that a degree of silence means things are not thought about or engaged is too simple. Absence of discussion does not mean a subject is absent from individual and social preoccupations (see Foucault, 1978). Reticence and euphemism may also be more complex phenomena than simply considering them as ipso facto evidence of a conspiracy of silence. They may capture a sensitivity about managing distress (Clow, 2001, p 302).

We can also question if silence always presupposes shame. It is clear that there have been many examples where people with cancer appear to be blamed for their disease. Sontag argues that patients who "are instructed that they have, unwittingly, caused their disease are also being made to feel that they have deserved it" (Sontag, 1991, p. 58). But these sorts of discursive constructions can prompt resistance. Clow cites a Gallup poll from 1950 where the question, "Do you think there is anything shameful in having cancer?" was answered "No" by 98% of those polled (Clow, 2001, p. 304).

CONTEMPORARY METAPHORS USED BY CLINICIANS

Froggatt studied U.K. nurses working in hospices, seeking to understand the place of metaphor in their emotional work. She identified "root metaphors": the "body as a container" and "emotions as energy" (Froggatt, 1998, p. 333). She attributes these to the resilience of the Cartesian split between mind and body, reason and emotion. The nurse's job becomes one of controlling the dangerous energy of emotions in themselves, their patients, and their patients' families. As nurses, they believed they had to "switch off" and "stand back." Emotional expression by patients "stirs up" or "rekindles" things. It risks being followed by the patients "breaking down." In addition to these fire metaphors, some emotions are described using water metaphors: floods of emotion bursting forth or a person being thrown overboard.

Sarbin argued that a person enters into a social role that can either be characterized as dramaturgical or dramatistic. "In a dramaturgical role, the individual consciously covers up any mismatch between what they feel and what they think they are meant to feel, using strategies of impression management, whereas when undertaking a dramatistic role the individual unconsciously takes on 'culturally available scripts,' for example the expectation of the expression of tears during a period of grief" (Sarbin, quoted in Froggatt, 1998, p. 336). Hockey (1993) applied this thesis to clergy undertaking funerals. Like Froggatt's hospice nurses, they display a root metaphor of the body as a container, and emotions as natural forces to be held within it. The clergy adopt a dramaturgical role as they consciously enact a social role at the funeral. Hospice nurses were dramatistic, their role influenced by "a complex mixture of judgments, values, intentions and acts, derived from various cultural sources" (Froggatt, 1998, p. 337).

Spall and colleagues (2001) ran focus groups with nurses, hospice staff, and bereavement counselors to identify the sources and functions of the metaphors they used. There is a sense here that these staff members are choosing narratives instrumentally, like Hockey's clergy. They consciously use metaphors as a way to help understanding, to facilitate communication, to educate. Sometimes they "co-construct" narratives with patients, taking the metaphors used by patients/clients and developing them. For example a nurse described how one patient's wife spoke proudly of how her husband was dealing with his illness by "put[ting] on a brave face." But she seemed to be having difficulty recognizing that he was now in the terminal phase of his condition. The nurse put it to her that, "He really has fought a good fight" and told how this metaphor "seemed to do something for her." Acknowledging his achievement seemed to let his wife accept what was happening (Spall et al., 2001, p. 347).

In all the professional groups reported in Spall et al., there were a significant number of metaphors that involved physical sensations: "being weighed down"; "frozen"; "I feel like there is a hole inside me"; "like walking around without any skin." All groups also used metaphors about travel, with hospice staff reporting the largest number: cancer as "a journey"; "traveling along a path." Bereavement counselors reported topographic metaphors, grief being described by clients as "like climbing a mountain." Discussions often included recognition of "peaks and troughs," of being "left dangling," of considerations about what can be "held on to." Other metaphors spoke of safety lines attached to others. One client described "feeling that she was tied to the point at which her husband had died by an elastic string, and no matter how far she went from it, she would always be pulled back." This form of words reassured Spall et al. because it seemed to be consistent with models of grief they recognized from the literature. These models, the Dual Process Model and the Continuing Bonds thesis, describe oscillations between loss and restoration orientations and the acceptability of continuing attachment to the dead person (Spall et al., 2001, p. 350; see also Stroebe & Schut, 1999; Klass et al., 1996).

Sontag reports on what she calls strenuous "conventions of concealment." "All this lying to and by cancer patients is a measure of how much harder it has become in advanced industrial societies to come to terms with death" (Sontag, 1991, pp. 7–8). But in the U.S. by the late 1970s, full disclosure of diagnosis was the norm. But even if diagnosis is now disclosed, research published in 2003 found continuing reluctance on the part of oncologists to discuss prognosis (Gordon & Daugherty, 2003), despite evidence that open discussion and knowledge of prognosis helps terminally ill patients and physicians better manage the death process in a way that reduces emotional distress (Christakis, 1999). Reluctance was expressed via two sorts of metaphor by oncologists. The first attributed it to a fear of the impact of prognosis on patients: "I don't want to hit someone in the face with it"; "I don't want to force it down their throats." The second sort of metaphor, by contrast, reflected a sense of the pressure patients had to exert to get the physician to disclose prognosis. The patient has to "really push you." In effect, the oncologist is shifting the responsibility for disclosure to the patient (Gordon & Daugherty, 2003, p. 156; see also DelVecchio Good, 1991).

In these interchanges, we can see a paradox in the contemporary discourse of cancer in the encounter between residual paternalism and self-determinism. Paternalism, evidenced by withholding information, is most often justified by a wish to preserve hope in the patient. Perhaps prognostic information will have what Christakis called "a prophecy effect" (1999). On the other hand, the prerequisite for self-determinism is timeliness and full disclosure. Engaging with this paradox requires analyzing our metaphors to help illuminate our implicit ethical and epistemological assumptions. Here, oncologists' metaphors of harm and of pressure present a complex picture of a vulnerable and demanding patient, unable to know their own best interests. It is "a paternalistic or protectionist approach to the relationship" (Gordon & Daugherty, 2003, p. 165). A shift to the partnership and patient-centered approach made possible by privileging autonomy and self-determination requires us to adopt new metaphors and new assumptions about the strengths and vulnerabilities of patients. Marshall and Koenig (1996) suggest that in approaches that assume a primacy for self-determinism, there is an "ideal patient," knowledgeable, future oriented, free to choose, and willing to discuss dying and death. This ideal patient well fits with the "reformist good death" that is aspired to by the hospice approach (Clark, 2002). This includes open acknowledgment, an aware death, resolution of both personal conflicts and unfinished business, and death according to personal preferences and in a manner that resonates with one's individuality.

Contemporary Metaphors: Patients

Gibbs and Franks (2002) studied in detail the metaphors used by six women in their narratives of cancer, cataloging 796 individual metaphors. Many could be grouped into metaphorical concepts and some were contradictory. Frequently occurring metaphorical concepts included "the body as a machine" and cancer as a war or battle. But the metaphorical concept most often used was that of a "journey." This concept is wider than illness. It is an organizing construct for thinking about one's life as a whole. Gibbs and Franks call this function "higher level mapping" (2002, p. 153). If your life is a journey, it implies a starting point, an ending, and a direction of travel. The journey is sometimes "diverted" or "derailed" by illness. "Cancer is an obstacle on life's journey"; "a bumpy road"; life is "at a crossroads." Cancer treatment becomes something "to get through." Journey metaphors can also present cancer as a place you travel into it and out of.

Kirmayer commented, "In sickness one confronts the inchoate. Bodily suffering disturbs the landscape of thought, rendering our previous construction incoherent and incomplete" (1992, p. 329). However, Gibbs and Franks demonstrate that the metaphors used by individuals with cancer show some continuity before and during their illness. The journey metaphor and embodied metaphors based on body sensations are sustained across changing circumstances.

Multiple metaphors, sometimes contradictory, are also not restricted to illness. If metaphors, as I have argued above, are not simply rhetorical devices, but contribute to meaning making and transmission, then complex and changing experiences may call up contradictory metaphors. Both the continuity of metaphor and its variety may have been underexamined in academic literature, including in Sontag's work, because of a focus on what could be termed the dramatic or poetic, consequently ignoring the wide range of conventional metaphors that characterize everyday speech. These are considered "dead" or "merely clichés" (Gibbs, 1994).

Gibbs and Franks examine a small group of people but there is also an increase in narratives of illness in the public domain. This increase was a steady one through the 1950s and 1960s, increasing in the 1990s and then in this century, there has been a huge growth, much of which is attributable to the Internet through narrative accounts of illness, web diaries, blogs, or contributions to web discussion groups (Little & Sayers, 2004; Pitts, 2004). There has also been an exponential increase in the way the Internet is used by people with cancer and by their caregivers to seek information and to access the experience of others (Ziebland, 2004).

Bingley et al. (2006) have sought to identify changes over time not just in the volume and location of narratives of illness, but also in the pattern of writing and the areas of concern engaged with. The areas most often referred to are stories of diagnosis, treatment and its impact, interactions with medicine, and the life outside the one bounded by medical encounters. It is the last of these that comes to increasing prominence in an approach to narrative that sees it as not just about speaking to others, but achieving a therapeutic benefit for the writer.

Arthur Frank (1995) sees three types of narratives in writings by those facing illness: narratives of restitution, chaos, and quest. His idea of there being story types is similar to the ideas of metaphors having some sort of hierarchical ordering, controlling metaphors or higher level metaphorical concepts, as described above. Narrators are "wounded storytellers." They shift their stance toward illness from a culturally prevalent passivity to activity. "The ill person who turns illness into story transforms fate into experience; the disease that sets the body apart from others becomes, in the story, the common bond of suffering that joins bodies in their shared vulnerability" (Frank, 1995, p. xi). Frank experienced life-threatening illness twice: a heart attack at 39 and cancer at 40. He writes, "Critical illness offers the experience of being taken to the threshold of life, from which you can see where your life could end" (Frank, 1991, p. 1). Telling his story is, for Frank, a survival kit, put together out of "a need to make sense of [his] own survival" (1995, p. xiii). But it is also an exemplar of what he believes about the times we live in: "Sooner or later, everyone is a wounded storyteller. In postmodern times that identity is our promise and responsibility, our calamity and dignity" (1995, p. xiii). We have, in Frank's work, military metaphors and journey metaphors and a strong sense of embodied experience. But we also have the sense of the possibility and potential of the person with cancer as an active agent using narrative in a way that is far from the shaming and silencing Sontag had attribute to a cancer diagnosis. Frank also is supportive of the idea of the subjectivity of postmodern times, the bitter challenge of having to make our selves.

Arthur Kleinman (1988) presents illness narratives, including those gathered from his experience as a clinician, as something from which we can all benefit. The journey metaphor is even more prevalent in his work. "We can envisage in chronic illness and its therapy a symbolic bridge that connects body, self and society. This network interconnects physiological processes, meanings and relationships so that our social world is linked recursively to our inner experience. Here we are privileged to discover powers within and between us that can either amplify suffering and disability or dampen symptoms and thereby contribute to care" (xiii-xiv).

CONCLUSIONS

A shift in the typical trajectory of cancer and in attitudes toward modernity means that cancer has lost some of its individual and social dread. A prevailing military metaphor, even if it existed when Sontag wrote, has been replaced by a multiplicity of metaphors. The military one remains but metaphors of choice and self-determinism, a shift characterized by journey metaphors, are increasing. Additionally, we need a much broader understanding of what function metaphor has. It is not just a rhetorical device for us to manipulate. Rather, it is inculcated in our semantic and epistemological selves.

In the brilliantly ironic opening page of *Illness as Metaphor* (Sontag, 1991, p. 3), Sontag seeks to effect a "mock exorcism of the seductiveness of metaphorical thinking" via writing "a brief hectic flourish of metaphor" (Sontag, 1991, p. 91). The metaphor she chooses is a journey one and her hectic flourish includes speaking of "a passport" to the different kingdoms of the well and of the sick. She speaks of "emigrating," "taking up residence," and of the lurid metaphors with which the kingdom of sick is "landscaped" (Sontag, 1991, p. 3). But in choosing a journey metaphor, she presages a more contemporary trope not just for illness, but for life. A journey metaphor, as developed in, for example, Frank and Kleinman, allows for recognition of agency both for the individual and for the conceptual and ontological use of metaphor itself. In this construction, "metaphors are as much a product of the lived experience of disease as they are a transforming influence on that experience" (Clow, 2001, p. 295). If some metaphors can lock you in enemy territory, others can be a key to help understand what is happening to you. They can be both oppressive and transformative.

ACKNOWLEDGMENT

I am grateful to Sherry Schachter at Calvary Hospital and Hospice in the Bronx, New York, for help with identifying literature relevant to contemporary uses of metaphor in engaging with cancer.

Neil Small *is a professor of health research at the University of Bradford, U.K. He is a sociologist who has a long-standing interest in chronic illness and end-of-life care. His recent focus has been on dementia and is reflected in the book* Living and Dying with Dementia: Dialogues about Palliative Care, *written with Katherine Froggatt and Murna Downs and published by Oxford University Press in 2007. In 2008 this book was named Medical Book of the Year (Non-Clinical), a prize awarded by the Royal Society of Medicine and the Society of Authors. His current work examines patterns of infant death and serious illness in the ethnically mixed and relatively deprived city of Bradford.*

REFERENCES

Bingley, A. F., McDermott, E., Thomas, C., Payne, S., Seymour, J. E., & Clark, D. (2006). Making sense of dying: A review of narratives written since 1950 by people facing death from cancer and other diseases. *Palliative Medicine, 20*, 183–195.

Christakis, N. (1999). *Death foretold: Prophecy and prognosis in medical care.* Chicago: University of Chicago Press.

Clark, D. (2002). Between hope and acceptance: The medicalisation of dying. *British Medical Journal, 324*, 905–907.

Clow, B. (2001). Who's afraid of Susan Sontag? Or, the myths and metaphors of cancer reconsidered. *Social History of Medicine, 14*(2), 293–312.

DelVecchio Good, M. J. (1991). The practice of biomedicine and the discourse on hope. *Anthropologies of Medicine, 7*, 121–135.

DiGiacomo, S. M. (1992). Metaphor as illness: Postmodern dilemmas in the representation of the body, mind and disorder. *Medical Anthropology, 14*, 109–37.

Foucault, M. (1973). *The birth of the clinic: An archaeology of medical perception.* London: Tavistock.

Foucault, M. (1978). *The history of sexuality.* London: Penguin.

Frank, A. (1991). *At the will of the body.* Boston: Mariner Books.

Frank, A. (1995). *The wounded storyteller.* Chicago: University of Chicago Press.

Froggatt, K. (1998). The place of metaphor and language in exploring nurses' emotional work. *Journal of Advanced Nursing, 28*(2), 332–338.

Gibbs, R. (1994). *The poetics of mind: Figurative thought, language and understanding*. New York: Cambridge University Press.

Gibbs Jr., R. W., & Franks, H. (2002). Embodied metaphor in women's narratives about their experiences with cancer. *Health Communication, 14*(2), 139–165.

Gordon, E. J., & Daugherty, C. K. (2003). Hitting you over the head: Oncologists' disclosure of prognosis to advanced cancer patients. *Bioethics, 17*(2), 142–168.

Hawkins, A. H. (1993). *Reconstructing illness: Studies in pathography*. West Lafayette, IN: Purdue University Press.

Hockey, J. (1993). The acceptable face of human grieving? In D. Clark (Ed.), *The sociology of death*, pp. 129–48. Oxford: Blackwell Science.

Kirmayer, L. (1992). The body's insistence on meaning: Metaphor as presentation and representation in illness experience. *Medical Anthropology Quarterly, 6*, 323–346.

Klass, D., Silverman, P., & Nickman, S. L. (1996). *Continuing bonds: New understandings of grief*. London: Taylor and Francis.

Kleinman, A. (1988). *The illness narratives*. New York: Basic Books.

Lakoff, G., & Johnson, M. (1980). *Metaphors we live by*. Chicago: Chicago University Press.

Lather, P. (2007). *Getting lost: Feminist efforts towards a double(d) science*. Albany, NY: State University of New York.

Little, M., & Sayers, E. J. (2004). While there's life...hope and the experience of cancer. *Social Science and Medicine, 59*, 1329–37.

Marshall, P. A., & Koenig, B. A. (1996). Bioethics in anthropology: Perspectives on culture, medicine and morality. In C. F. Sargent, & T. F. Johnson (Eds.), *Medical anthropology: Contemporary theory and method*, Revised Edition, pp. 349–373. Westport, CT: Praeger.

Patterson, J. T. (1987). *The dread disease: Cancer and modern American culture*. Cambridge, MA: Harvard University Press.

Pitts, V. (2004). Illness and Internet empowerment: Writing and reading breast cancer in cyberspace. *Health, 8*, 33–59.

Ricoeur, P. (1986). *The rule of metaphor: Multi-disciplinary studies in the creation of meaning.* London: Routledge and Kegan Paul.

Sarbin, T. R. (1986). Emotion and act: Roles and rhetoric. In R. Harre (Ed.), *The social construction of emotions,* pp. 83–97. Oxford: Basil Blackwell.

Sontag, S. (1991). *Illness as metaphor and AIDS and its metaphors.* London: Penguin.

Spall, B., Read, S., & Chantry, D. (2001). Metaphor: Exploring its origins and therapeutic use in death, dying and bereavement. *International Journal of Palliative Nursing, 7*(7), 345–353.

Stacey, J. (1997). *Teratologies: A cultural study of cancer.* London: Routledge.

Stroebe, M., & Schut, H. (1999). The dual process model of coping with bereavement: Rationale and description. *Death Studies, 23,* 197–224.

Ziebland, S. (2004). The importance of being expert: The quest for cancer information on the Internet. *Social Science and Medicine, 59,* 1783–93.

Treating Cancer

Throughout the past 75 years, there have been remarkable strides in cancer treatment. Brad Stuart begins this section with an overview, essentially a primer on available options including surgery, chemotherapy, radiation therapy, and targeted therapies. Stuart's review reaffirms two critical points. Cancer treatment is generally most effective when the cancer is confined to one organ or a localized area and when the whole cancerous mass can be removed. Stuart's second point is also essential: When cancer has become advanced, referrals to palliative care and hospice should be assessed early enough so patients can benefit from these modalities.

As Doka indicated in the opening chapter, there has always existed, along with conventional treatment, unconventional options. Lynda Shand's chapter deals with complementary or alternative medicine (CAM). As Shand notes, the often-made distinction that alternative therapies are used *instead* of conventional medicine while complementary therapies are used *along with* conventional medicine is sometimes more fluid than thought. In addition, Shand recognizes that patients frequently revert to complementary or alternative medicine since they offer both hope and control. She importantly suggests that physicians treating patients should routinely assess patients' use of CAM therapies. This will become even more essential as the Baby Boom generation ages because hope and, especially, control are generational values for this Internet-savvy cohort.

Advances in the treatment of cancer have created many gray areas where, as Nancy Berlinger and Bruce Jennings contend, ethical dilemmas abound. These areas include places where sharp distinctions such as between treatment and research, between therapeutic treatment and palliative treatment, between hospital and hospice, between the process of living with a chronic illness and the process of dying from a progressive illness have become blurred. The culture of cancer, the authors assert, is still a culture where the goal is cure. Yet, the reality is that for many patients, they are living with a chronic, even progressive disease. Berlinger and Jennings affirm that communication and collaboration, as well as flexibility between institutions and policies, provide space for managing the "thin places" between these ever-changing boundaries.

In "The Transition to Palliative Care" Brad Stuart not only draws on his prior chapter but also complements the writings of Shand, and Berlinger and Jennings. Stuart is sensitive to the fact that the transition to palliative care is not only a medical one; it is primarily an emotional one. Facing life's end, humans—whether patients, families, or physicians—are rarely totally rational. Many prefer continued therapy, even futile treatments, as it is seen as "doing something." Stuart offers sensitive guidelines for managing that transition. These guidelines suggest again that communication and collaboration are essential in managing to balance hope and reality.

Sherry Schachter's chapter offers an apt ending for this section. Using both theory and case studies, Schachter describes the nature of good end-of-life care, emphasizing that it is inherently holistic: encompassing not only excellent medical care, but also concern for the ethical dimensions of care and recognition of the value of psychosocial, spiritual, and existential concern. Schachter's work emphasizes the importance of continuity of care. It is critical that patients do not feel abandoned by their families, friends, physicians, and faith community. Even when patients make the transition to end-of-life care, from cure to comfort, they need not do it alone.

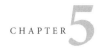

Treatment Options in Cancer

Brad Stuart

A diagnosis of cancer brings with it a host of decisions for clinicians, patients, and families. The probability of cure depends on the type of cancer, i.e., its organ of primary origin and whether it is still confined to this site or has already spread beyond it at the time of diagnosis. Even when cancer has spread, either by direct invasion of neighboring structures or metastasis via the bloodstream or the lymphatic system, it may still be controllable with treatment even if it cannot be cured. Therefore, it is important to obtain a thorough assessment by a qualified physician, usually an oncologist, who can then recommend a treatment plan.

Depending on the tumor type, there may be a range of treatment options that patients and families, with physician guidance, may choose from. Some cancers can be treated in several ways. Prostate cancer still confined to the gland, for example, is curable through surgery, i.e., radical prostatectomy; with radiation therapy, which can be administered locally through implantation of radioactive "seeds" directly into the prostate gland; or through external beam radiotherapy. Patients and families can discuss these choices with a urologic surgeon and a radiation oncologist to decide which treatment regimen suits them best. Many cancer centers have both kinds of specialists available for consultation to aid informed decisions.

Cancer treatment is provided through several modalities. The most common are surgery, chemotherapy, radiation therapy, targeted therapy, and palliative care. Each has its specific indications, and several may be used in combination. This paper describes each in turn, ideally providing enough detail to allow nonphysicians to feel comfortable with making decisions about cancer treatment in collaboration with their clinicians.

Many cancers cause bothersome symptoms as they progress. In particular, pain can be associated with both metastatic cancer and its treatment. Also, not all cancers are curable. Many have spread to other parts of the body before they produced enough symptoms to trigger physician evaluation. Others have progressed beyond curable stages despite treatment. For these reasons, palliative care, or treatment focused on the patient's comfort rather than on cure, has recently assumed greater importance in cancer care. Although some people may confuse palliative care with end-of-life care, the two are distinct. Palliative care may be indicated at any stage of cancer treatment, usually to treat unpleasant symptoms or to help patients and families with difficult choices, for example, weighing burdens vs. benefits of further treatment in advanced disease. Many cancer centers provide specialized palliative care right along with cancer treatment.

Hospice is the subset of palliative care that applies most appropriately when patients begin to approach the end of life. However, prognosis, or the determination of how long a cancer patient might live, is not an exact science. Also, hospice has been shown to actually extend life in most types of cancer compared with usual care (Connor, Pyenson, Fitch, Spence, & Iwasake, 2007). To make sure patients get the best symptom management and support, early referral to hospice should be considered when cancer becomes advanced.

SURGERY

Surgical removal of cancerous tissue was the first form of cancer treatment. Surgical techniques continue to advance. Minimally invasive surgery, e.g., through an endoscope, can help to preserve normal tissue and function.

Patients usually undergo a surgical biopsy to confirm a cancer diagnosis. Tissue specimens are typically submitted for pathological analysis under a microscope using special stains. This is critical to determine the cancer tissue type and to decide on the most effective treatment regimen. Surgical staging employing procedures like laparotomy (surgical exploration of the abdomen) or laparoscopy (abdominal exploration through an endoscope) can help to determine the extent to which the cancer has spread and, in turn, to formulate the most accurate prognosis and treatment plan.

Surgery can be curative when cancer is confined to one organ or localized area and when it appears likely that all malignant tissue can be removed during the procedure. When cancer is too widespread for total excision, surgical debulking can remove major parts of the tumor mass while avoiding damage to uninvolved tissues. Chemotherapy or radiation may then be used to treat any remaining cancerous tissue. Palliative surgery in advanced cases can remove tumors that are causing uncomfortable complications, e.g., blockage of airways or intestines. Finally, reconstructive surgery, e.g., of the breast after mastectomy, can restore normal function or appearance after major cancer surgery.

CHEMOTHERAPY

Although there are many types of cancer, they all have in common malignant changes in cell structure, causing rapid and uncontrolled growth. Cytotoxic chemotherapy, which has been used in cancer care since the 1950s, attacks and kills rapidly dividing cells. Like surgery, it can be used to cure, control, or palliate cancer. Most oncologists use the word "cure" cautiously, because it takes time, usually five years or more, to be sure that the cancer was fully eradicated and will not recur.

Chemotherapy is often administered intravenously (by vein), but it can also be given intramuscularly (injection into muscle) or by mouth. It can be given alone, as neoadjuvant therapy (before surgery or radiation), or as adjuvant therapy (after surgery or radiation). The drugs mentioned in this section are directly toxic to cells; they should be distinguished from "targeted therapy" drugs discussed later in this paper.

Because cytotoxic chemotherapy kills all cells that divide rapidly, cancerous or not, it can cause side effects by damaging body systems that need to regenerate constantly to stay healthy. Common side effects from chemotherapy thus include hair loss; bone marrow suppression (eliminating white cells that fight infection, platelets that help with blood clotting, and red cells that carry oxygen to tissues); gastrointestinal upset due to damage of the lining of stomach and intestines; and mouth sores. Medication and other treatments are available to prevent or ameliorate many of these side effects. Chemotherapy can also adversely affect sexual function and reproductive ability.

Chemotherapy drugs fall into several classes based on their chemical structures or mechanisms of action. Drugs from several different classes may be used together in the same treatment regimen based on results of clinical trials. Side effects are often similar among drugs in the same class. Common types of chemotherapeutic agents (listed by generic name) include the following:

- *Alkylating agents*: These drugs attack DNA to prevent cell reproduction. They can produce bone marrow damage in survivors, which can result in dose-dependent leukemias that are most commonly seen 5 to 10 years after treatment. Subclasses of alkylating agents include
  - *Nitrogen mustards*: mechlorethamine, chlorambucil, cyclophosphamide
  - *Nitrosoureas*: streptozocin, carmustine, lomustine
  - *Alkyl sulfonates*: busulfan
  - *Triazines*: procarbazine, dacarbazine, temozolomide
  - *Ethylenimines*: thioTEPA, altretamine

- *Platinum-based drugs*: These drugs also kill cells through DNA damage, but they are less likely to cause secondary leukemias. Examples include cisplatin, carboplatin, and oxaliplatin.
- *Antimetabolites*: These drugs interfere with DNA and RNA synthesis by substituting other building blocks for the normal structures of these genetic molecules. Examples include methotrexate, 5-fluorouracil, cytarabine, fludarabine, 6-mercaptopurine, gemcitabine, capecitabine, and pemetrexed.
- *Anthracyclines*: These drugs interfere with enzymes that help with DNA replication and are widely used for many types of cancers. They can damage the heart muscle above a certain total threshold dose, which should not be exceeded in the patient's lifetime. Examples include doxorubicin, daunorubicin, epirubicin, and idarubicin.
- *Antitumor antibiotics*: These include actinomycin-D, mitomycin-C, bleomycin, and plicamycin.
- *Topoisomerase I and II inhibitors*: These drugs block enzymes that separate DNA strands for copying. Topoisomerase I inhibitors include topotecan and irinotecan. Topoisomerase II inhibitors, which can cause secondary leukemias within 2 to 3 years of administration, include etoposide (VP-16), teniposide, and mitoxantrone.
- *Mitotic inhibitors*: These drugs, many of which are derived from plants, interfere with cell division. They can damage nerves in hands and feet, causing painful neuropathies that often limit treatment. Subclasses include
  - *Vinca alkaloids*: vincristine, vinblastine, vinorelbine
  - *Taxanes*: paclitaxel, docetaxel
  - *Epothilones*: ixabepilone
- *Corticosteroids*: These are natural hormones or synthetic analogues that are useful in treating certain cancers. Examples include prednisone, dexamethasone, and methylprednisolone. These drugs are also used to treat side effects of other drugs and symptoms of cancer itself, especially nausea and vomiting.
- *Other chemotherapeutic agents*: These do not fit into the listed categories, or their indications are limited to a small number of tumors.

RADIATION THERAPY

X-rays and other forms of ionizing radiation form ions, or electrically charged particles, in cells they pass through, damaging or killing them. Microwaves, radio waves, and light waves are of lower energy and thus don't produce cell damage. Radiation is used for local treatment of cancer; it is not indicated for malignancies that have spread throughout the body. Radiation therapy kills tumor cells, but it also damages normal tissues that are also penetrated by the radiation in front of and behind the tumor. Therefore, careful treatment planning is necessary, using detailed imaging studies and computer dose calculations, prior to beginning therapy. Radiation therapy is usually given in daily fractions over a period of several weeks.

Radiation therapy can sometimes cure early-stage cancer that is confined to one area, or at least reduce tumor size. Cancer recurrence can be prevented in areas where tumor cells have a high probability of causing future problems. For example, whole-brain radiation is often employed in lung cancer to prevent brain metastases. Finally, palliative radiation can reduce symptoms such as shortness of breath from tumor obstruction of an airway, or pain resulting from cancer growth into a major nerve. Palliative radiation can be given in just one or two large fractions to rapidly maximize treatment effects and to promote comfort.

The most common radiation used in cancer treatment is in the form of high-energy photon beams emitted from radioactive cobalt or cesium. These may also be produced in a linear accelerator, which can also provide electron beams of lower energy. Higher-energy radiation penetrates to deep structures, while electron beam therapy is used to treat tumors close to the skin. Proton beam therapy—still under study and not yet widely available—may kill tumor cells at the end of its track but produce less damage as it travels through normal tissue. However, proton sources can also expose patients to neutrons, which can cause severe long-term side effects.

Brachytherapy (radiation treatment over short distances, often fractions of an inch) is useful for tumors that require high doses of radiation that would damage over- and underlying tissues if a beam were used. Brachytherapy is administered interstitially, through implantation of pellets, or via intracavitary radiation through placement of a container of radioactive material in the chest, uterus, or vagina. Permanent brachytherapy, used to treat prostate cancer, for example, usually entails implantation of seeds or pellets with short radioactive decay times that are left in place. Temporary brachytherapy, either high or low dose, involves placing needles or tubes in or near the tumor, filling them with radioactive substance for a defined period of time, and withdrawing them. Because precise placement of radioactive material needs to be maintained throughout treatment, brachytherapy may require hospitalization.

TARGETED THERAPY

Targeted therapy, a relatively recent innovation, attacks cancer cells selectively while leaving healthy cells in the bone marrow and intestines relatively unharmed. These drugs take advantage of new knowledge about the biochemistry and physiology of cancer cells, focusing on molecular mechanisms unique to them. Targeted therapy disrupts intracellular processes that maintain malignant cell proliferation, repair, and spread. Much current research is concentrated on this field, and advances can be expected as new discoveries occur.

Targeted therapies tend not to be curative, but they can slow or reverse the growth and spread of some cancers. They can be used alone or in combination with cytotoxic chemotherapy or radiation (Ma & Waxman, 2008). They fall into several categories, based on their mechanisms of action. Many are small-molecule enzyme or signal-transduction inhibitors that block the action of metabolic steps that are critical to cancer cells. Others induce apoptosis, or programmed cell death, by changing proteins that are necessary for survival of cancer cells. Others inhibit angiogenesis, or the growth of blood vessels bringing circulation to tumors, by blocking vascular endothelial growth factor. Because the list of available targeted drugs is long and constantly evolving, they will not be listed here.

PALLIATIVE CARE

Many patients experience troublesome symptoms as their disease advances. For example, most cancer patients eventually have pain severe enough to prevent going to work or pursuing normal activity. Accordingly, palliative care has become an important component of cancer treatment. Palliative care is defined by the World Health Organization (WHO) (2005) as "an approach that improves the quality of life of patients and their families facing the problem associated with life-threatening illness, through the prevention and relief of suffering by means of early identification and impeccable assessment and treatment of pain and other problems, physical, psychosocial and spiritual." Although a description of the entire field of palliative care is beyond the scope of this paper, the basics of pain management in cancer are outlined here, with emphasis on oral treatment that is usually effective even in the most severe cases of cancer pain and can be given easily and safely at home. Common brand names are given to help identify analgesic drugs, although generic equivalents are available for most of them.

Cancer pain falls into three broad categories: somatic, visceral, and neuropathic. Somatic pain results from damage to bone, muscle, and other tissues. It is usually easy for patients to localize, often by pointing a finger. Its character can be dull or sharp, but patients can usually describe it easily. Visceral pain, usually located in the abdomen, is caused by damage to organs in and around the digestive tract. It may be dull or crampy and can radiate to other parts of the abdomen or to the back. Neuropathic pain, resulting from damage to nerve tracts or to the spine or brain, can be harder to describe and therefore to diagnose, and it is often missed. It can have a shooting or burning character and often radiates down the distribution of the nerve. Cancer pain that requires high doses of opioid analgesics or that responds poorly to such treatment may be neuropathic in origin.

The WHO analgesic ladder is a stepwise approach that can guide analgesic treatment (World Health Organization, 2009). Pain that is mild, or rated by the patient as 1–3 on a scale of 10, may respond to nonopioid analgesics like aspirin, acetaminophen, or nonsteroidal antiinflammatory drugs (NSAIDs). Moderate pain of 3–5 out of 10 may be treated with weak opioids such as combinations of hydrocodone and acetaminophen (Norco®, Vicodin®). Codeine, also classified as a weak opioid, is usually prescribed in combination with acetaminophen, although it has a higher incidence of side effects like nausea and dysphoria, an unpleasant or depressive emotional state. Recently, the U.S. Food and Drug Administration (FDA) has focused attention on these drugs because of their easy availability and addictive potential when prescribed for noncancer chronic pain. Moreover, the acetaminophen component is toxic to the liver in high doses, and some patients may take more of the drug as their pain increases, as it tends to do as cancer advances. Consequently, moderate cancer pain may be treated just as effectively, and perhaps more safely, with strong opioids alone.

The strong opioids most commonly used in the United States are morphine, oxycodone, hydromorphone (Dilaudid®), and methadone. Any of these drugs may be given through several routes of administration, e.g., orally, sublingually (under the tongue), intramuscularly, subcutaneously (through a needle implanted beneath the skin, often using an automatic pump), or intravenously (IV). It is important to emphasize, however, that almost all cases of cancer pain, even the most severe, can be treated with opioids given by mouth (Bruera & Kim, 2003). Decades of experience in hospice care have shown that patients discharged from the hospital on IV morphine, for example, can be converted easily and safely to oral morphine at home.

The most widely available opioid for cancer pain management is an oral solution of morphine sulfate instant-release (MSIR) at the concentration of 20 mg/ml (Roxanol®). One milliliter (ml) equals 1/5 of a teaspoon. A starting dose of 5 mg of morphine, about equivalent in potency to one Vicodin® tablet, amounts to 1/4 ml, or 1/20th of a teaspoon. This means that an effective dose of morphine can be delivered in a very small volume of liquid, and the dosage can easily be adjusted upward if pain worsens. This approach works well for patients with severe pain who have difficulty swallowing, as often happens in late-stage cancer. MSIR also relieves shortness of breath (dyspnea) in patients with diseases like lung cancer or chronic lung disease (Jennings, Davies, Higgins, Gibbs, & Broadley, 2002).

The onset of pain relief after taking oral morphine is 30–60 minutes, and a single dose lasts for up to 4 hours. Cancer pain is most effectively treated by giving morphine every 4 hours around the clock. Staying ahead of the pain this way actually requires less medication than waiting for pain to recur before giving the next dose.

When patients require around-the-clock dosing, however, it is often more convenient to switch to morphine sulfate sustained-release (MSSR) in pill form (MS Contin®). This long-acting form of morphine, available in many different dosages, can be given every 12 hours in most cases. Conversion to MSSR is accomplished by calculating the 24-hour total required MSIR dose, then splitting it in half and giving the closest available MSSR dose. MSIR should also be made available, however, for incidents of sudden "breakthrough pain" or to supplement MSSR doses if the baseline level of cancer pain increases. MSIR breakthrough doses, usually set at about one third of the 12-hour MSSR dose, can be given at intervals as short as 1 hour apart for pain crises until adequate analgesia is restored. Then the MSSR dose can be adjusted upward, and the MSIR breakthrough dose recalculated to one third of the MSSR dose.

Adjusting the morphine dose to a higher level, also known as upward dose titration, is usually necessary as the disease advances. A common rule of thumb in cancer pain management is "start low, go slow." Initial doses adequate to control pain should be provided and titrated upward just rapidly enough to get pain under control and keep it that way. Too high an initial dose or overly rapid dosage titration can result in toxicity, most commonly manifested as drowsiness, confusion, or other signs of oversedation. Potentially lethal complications, e.g., suppression of respiration, are uncommon with a cautious approach even in cases where severe lung disease is present. Non-life-threatening oversedation can be managed simply by withholding morphine doses just until the patient returns to a more normal level of consciousness, then restarting morphine at a lower dose. Opioid antagonists, e.g., naloxone (Narcan®), are rarely necessary unless spontaneous breathing is compromised.

It is important to note, however, that patients with severe pain may require very high doses of morphine, and sometimes sedative medication, to keep symptoms under control (Moryl, Coyle, & Foley, 2008), if all other interventions, e.g., nerve block (Wong et al., 2004), have failed. It is distressing to family members, and unfortunately common especially in hospitals, for clinicians to withhold morphine and sedatives for fear of suppressing respiration, only to have the patient die with untreated pain and shortness of breath. This is an issue of quality care that palliative care clinicians are attempting to address, with some success.

From an ethical and legal standpoint, relief of distressing symptoms in dying patients is a clinical imperative, even if there is fear life may be shortened. This kind of treatment should not be mistaken for assisted suicide or euthanasia, because the primary intent is to manage symptoms, not to cause the patient to die. Recent studies show that even aggressive treatment with opioids and sedatives does not, in fact, hasten death (Sykes & Thorns, 2003).

For most patients, morphine in its short- and long-acting forms works well to control cancer pain. Transient side effects, e.g., dizziness or nausea, can be managed conservatively or with other medications and usually pass after a day or two. True allergy to morphine—manifested by skin rash, hives, wheezing, or other allergic symptoms—is uncommon. A few patients really cannot tolerate morphine, most commonly when it causes hallucinations. Also, some patients on large doses of morphine for long periods of time, especially those with poor kidney function, can develop neurotoxic side effects, probably due to the accumulation of toxic byproducts from liver metabolism of morphine. Excitability may occur, or even paradoxical pain that becomes worse with higher morphine doses. Opioid rotation, or conversion of the analgesic regimen to another opioid, e.g., methadone, is then indicated (Crews, Sweeney, & Denson, 1993).

Oxycodone is also available in IR (OxyFast®, OxyIR®) or SR (Oxycontin®) forms. Because it is about 1.5 times more potent than morphine in its analgesic effect, and because of its potential for sedation if too high a dose is used, conversion from morphine to oxycodone requires a reduction in dose by a factor of 1.5. For example, a patient taking 300 mg of morphine a day (doses this high are commonly required in patients with advanced cancer) could be started on oxycodone SR 100 mg every 12 hours, for a total of 200 mg/day. Oxycodone IR should also be provided for breakthrough pain.

Hydromorphone is available only in IR form; an SR preparation has not been approved for use in the United States. Hydromorphone is shorter acting than morphine, so its required dosage interval may be as short as 2–3 hours in some cases. This makes the drug somewhat less practical for management of chronic cancer pain than morphine and oxycodone. In addition, hydromorphone may have higher abuse potential than other opioids.

Methadone, a synthetic opioid, deserves special mention because of its unique properties and low cost. Developed around World War II, methadone acts on opioid receptors in a manner similar to other opioids, but it also activates neurons in the spinal cord that slow the transmission of pain impulses to the brain. This may be why methadone appears to be more effective in the treatment of neuropathic pain than are morphine and other opioids (Watanabe, 2001). Methadone is absorbed through oral mucous membranes at higher rates than morphine, so liquid methadone may be useful in cases where patients lose the ability to swallow, as often occurs near death. The drug is intrinsically long acting, so no SR preparation is necessary. However, because methadone's persistence in the bloodstream is so long, and also because the length of time varies unpredictably from patient to patient, caution is needed when starting patients on methadone. The drug may accumulate over several days, causing sedation and respiratory failure if the patient is not carefully observed.

CONCLUSION

Many options are available for the treatment of cancer. The disease is often curable when it is caught before it spreads beyond its organ of origin. Even if metastasis has occurred, however, treatment may slow its growth. When symptoms like pain occur, or when the disease becomes advanced, palliative care and hospice should be accessed, and referral should be made early enough that the patient gains maximal benefit.

Brad Stuart, MD, was the primary author of Medical Guidelines for Prognosis in Selected Non-Cancer Diseases, *adopted as national Medicare hospice eligibility criteria. He has received the Heart of Hospice Award from the National Hospice and Palliative Care Organization, and the California State Hospice Association's Pierre Salmon Award. In 2007 he was voted "Physician of the Year" by the California Association for Health Services at Home. Dr. Stuart was featured in the HBO documentary* Letting Go: A Hospice Journey, *and has been interviewed on NBC's* Good Morning America. *He wrote and hosted* Care Beyond Cure: Hospice Helping Physicians Treat the Terminally Ill, *a nationally televised Continuing Medical Education video that won an International Angel Award for Media Excellence. He has published widely and lectured internationally on medical, psychosocial, and spiritual issues at the end of life.*

REFERENCES

Bruera, E., & Kim, H. N. (2003). Cancer pain. *JAMA, 290,* 2476–2479.

Connor, S. R., Pyenson, B., Fitch, K., Spence, C., & Iwasake, K. (2007). Comparing hospice and non-hospice patient survival among patients who die within a three-year window. *Journal of Pain and Symptom Management, 33,* 238–246.

Crews, J. C., Sweeney, N. J., & Denson, D. D. (1993). Clinical efficacy of methadone in patients refractory to other μ-opioid receptor agonist analgesics for management of terminal cancer pain. *Cancer, 72,* 2266–2272.

Jennings, A. L., Davies, A. N., Higgins, J. P. T., Gibbs, J. S. R., & Broadley, K. E. (2002). A systematic review of the use of opioids in the management of dyspnea. *Thorax, 57,* 939–944.

Ma, J., & Waxman, D. J. (2008). Combination of antiangiogenesis with chemotherapy for more effective cancer treatment. *Molecular Cancer Therapeutics, 7,* 3670–3684.

Moryl, N. M., Coyle, N., & Foley, K. M. (2008). Managing an acute pain crisis in a patient with advanced cancer. *JAMA, 299,* 1457–1467.

Sykes, N., & Thorns, A. (2003). The use of opioids and sedatives at end of life. *The Lancet Oncology, 4,* 312–318.

Watanabe, S. (2001). Methadone: The renaissance. *Journal of Palliative Care, 17,* 117–120.

Wong, G. Y., Schroeder, D. R., Carns, P. E., Wilson, J. L., Martin, D. P., Kinney, M. O., et al. (2004). Effect of neurolytic celiac plexus block on pain relief, quality of life, and survival in patients with unresectable pancreatic cancer. *JAMA, 291*, 1092–1099.

World Health Organization. (2005). WHO definition of palliative care. Retrieved July 30, 2009, from http://www.who.int/cancer/palliative/definition/en

World Health Organization. (2009). WHO pain ladder. Retrieved July 30, 2009, from http://www.who.int/cancer/palliative/painladder/en/

CHAPTER 6

Complementary and Alternative Cancer Therapies: Don't Ask, Don't Tell

Lynda Shand

M ore than a million adults in the United States had some form of cancer in 2008 (American Cancer Society, n.d.). Great progress has been made in treatment, including chemotherapy and radiation. However, this conventional treatment often targets the disease process and overlooks the whole person. A patient told me, "I want my cancer treated by the best oncologists, that's why I am here at the Center. But I also want to be listened to, be part of the decision-making process. I want my well-being attended to, not just my cancer."

The increasing popularity and use of complementary or alternative medicine (CAM) therapies in the general population and among cancer patients has been well documented in scientific literature and published in popular literature (Austin, 1998; Cassileth, Schraub, Robinson, & Vickers, 2001; Chatwin & Tovey, 2004; Molassiotis et al., 2005; Ott, 2002; Peace & Manesse, 2002). Estimates of CAM use vary widely depending on the definition and sampling strategies utilized. However, a study by Barnes, Powell-Griner, McFann, and Nahin (2004) revealed that 75% of the representative sample used CAM at some time in their lives for health reasons. There are now more healthcare facilities providing CAM therapies and insurance companies offering reimbursement for these products and services.

More than ever before, people often choose one or more nontraditional products or practices after they are diagnosed with cancer (Jordan & Delunas, 2001), and more than one-third of the general population of the United States reports using CAM (Sparber et al., 2000). A study conducted by Eisenberg et al. (1998) revealed that one in three respondents reported using at least one CAM therapy in the past year, and a third of these saw providers for unconventional therapy. Ernst and Cassileth (1998) conducted a systematic review and reported CAM use among adult patients with cancer to be between 7% and 64%. This was also reflected in the study by Fouladbakhsh, Stommel, Given, and Given (2005), who found that nearly 30% of the participants used CAM therapy.

Cancer patients want more information on CAM therapies and access to CAM products and practitioners. Many believe CAM therapies should be offered as part of conventional treatment protocols (Mao, Farrar, Xie, Bowman, & Armstrong, 2007). Healthcare practitioners (HCPs) and members of the interdisciplinary care team who do not discuss CAM with patients lose an opportunity to explore patients' unmet needs as well as establish an informed discussion of effects and interactions.

WHAT IS CAM?

There are many terms used to describe approaches to healing and health restoration that are considered outside the realm of conventional medicine as practiced in the United States. There is no consensus on terminology used to describe complementary and alternative health practices. Eisenberg et al. (1993) described CAM therapies as all therapies not routinely taught at U.S. medical schools and not routinely available at U.S. hospitals. The M. D. Anderson Cancer Center Web site refers to complementary therapies as those that complement conventional therapies, and alternative medicine as therapeutic approaches that take the place of conventional medicines or protocols used to treat disease (M. D. Anderson Cancer Center, n.d.).

For our purposes here, let us consider CAM therapies as they are defined by the National Center for Complementary and Alternative Medicine (NCCAM): a group of diverse medical and healthcare systems, practices, and products that are not presently considered to be part of conventional medicine. According to NCCAM, "The list of practices that are considered CAM changes continually as CAM practices and therapies that are proven safe and effective become accepted as 'mainstream healthcare practices.'" The Web site (http://nccam.nih.gov/health/whatiscam/overview.htm) details what NCCAM considers the five major domains of CAM: (1) "whole medical systems" such as homeopathic and Chinese medicine; (2) "mind-body medicine" such as meditation, support groups, prayer, and dance; (3) "biologically based practices" such as herbal products, dietary supplements, foods, and vitamins; (4) "manipulative and body-based practices" such as chiropractic medicine, massage, and naturopathy; and (5) "energy medicine" such as Reiki, therapeutic touch, and electromagnetic fields.

A detailed review of CAM products and practices is not the goal of this paper. Instead, this paper presents an overview of studies that examine use of CAM therapies by people with cancer as well as counseling implications.

WHY PATIENTS TURN TO CAM

Although patients are attracted to CAM therapies for a variety of reasons, the most frequently cited reason for patients to seek CAM therapies is to relieve the side effects of cancer treatment or symptoms of cancer. A National Institutes of Health Consensus Conference (1998) reported evidence that supports the efficacy of acupuncture in relieving chemotherapy-related nausea and vomiting. Several randomized controlled studies support the use of psychological and mind-body therapies to relieve cancer-related pain (Sloman, Brown, Aldana, & Chee, 1994; Syrjala, Donaldson, Davis, Kippes, & Carr, 1995).

Elliot, Kealey, and Oliver (2008) reported on patients using CAM therapies for perceived physical, psychological, philosophical, and social benefits as well as a more holistic approach to cancer treatment. Other individuals, with active coping styles, seek CAM therapies to help feel in control, referring to CAM as something they can do for themselves (Humpel, 2006; Sollner et al., 2000). Patients studied by Correa-Velez, Clavino, and Eastwood (2005) used CAM therapies as complementary to rather than as an alternative to conventional cancer treatment. This group reported side effects from traditional cancer treatments and used CAM therapies to detoxify their bodies and boost immunity to "prolong their survival, palliate their symptoms or alleviate them, and enhance their overall quality of life" (p. 953).

A patient in our practice was forced to withdraw from a clinical trial due to disease progression, an exclusion factor for continued participation. The patient was distraught as she felt this clinical trial was her "last hope." Several weeks later she was admitted to the Center with severe bleeding that appeared to be unrelated to either her disease progression or prescribed treatment. After a long and tearful discussion, the patient confided that she "went on line" to find something to "slow the cancer and save my life." The herbal remedy she was using had depleted the ability of her blood to clot. Patients' use of CAM therapies may not be based on scientific evidence but rather on hope. She said, "I needed to do *something!*"

"While there are well-documented therapies that augment cancer treatment and minimize side effects of chemotherapy and radiation, there are also products and practices that can harm patients either by disrupting effective cancer treatment or directly inflicting physiologic harm" (Marshall, 2001, para. 1). Many patients believe herbal products are better because they are natural. The use of "natural products" may result in unexpected and dangerous side effects if the patient initiates CAM therapies without a discussion with the HCP or a certified CAM practitioner. CAM use by a patient acting alone may result in undesirable and unexpected effects due to lack of product regulation, incomplete or misleading dosing information, uninformed decision making, or delay of conventional treatment. It is likely that many practitioners have in their practices patients who are using undisclosed CAM therapies. Use of CAM therapies may remain unreported by patients unless, like our patient, they present with unusual symptoms, complaints, or unexpected side effects. Patients are unsure if they should tell, and HCPs do not ask. What is lost is an opportunity to collaborate and discuss what works, what does not, and what can be harmful.

The use of CAM therapies is often not discussed openly between patients and caregivers (Adler & Fosket, 1999; Eisenberg et al., 1993; Evans et al., 2007; Gray et al., 1997). Less than 40% of patients discuss CAM with their HCPs (Eisenberg et al, 1998). Rather, they rely on popular magazines, books, newspapers, the Internet, television, and television personalities for information. As a result, patients are exposed to the promises of a wide variety of practices and products, most unevaluated by clinical trial. The hope for relief of symptoms or a cure may lead patients to risk untested and unregulated remedies.

HCPs need greater awareness of the reasons for and the nature of patients' choices. When the use of CAM is disclosed, HCPs can work with patients to help them make informed and medically safe choices. Early, open discussions should focus on the individual patient's needs, goals, and hopes with sensitivity to cultural and religious beliefs.

WHY PATIENTS DO NOT TELL

Patients are reticent to openly communicate the use of CAM therapies if they perceive "…indifference or opposition toward CAM use; physician's emphasis on scientific evidence; and [patient's] anticipation of a negative response from the physician" (Tasaki, Maskarinec, Shumay, Tatsumura, & Kakai, 2002, p. 214). Other patients are apprehensive of their HCPs' reaction or fearful of disapproval (Coss, McGrath, & Caggiano, 1998; Michaud, 2000). A patient was asked why she did not tell the oncologist about the extensive list of vitamins, herbs, and magnets she used to control symptoms and "fight the cancer." She said, "He would only tell me I was crazy!"

During a clinic visit, when a new patient to our service was asked why he did not add CAM use to his health history, he replied, "No one ever asked. You're the first." Another said, "When you only have a short time with the doc, most of the things she is concerned with are attended to first. You run out of time, they run out of time." Wynia, Eisenberg, and Wilson (1999) found "that having sufficient time during patient visits (visit length) would be correlated with the frequency with which physicians discussed CAM therapies with patients" (p. 448).

WHY HCPs DO NOT ASK

Gray et al. (1997) reported that few physicians in the study stated they would discuss CAM with their patients. For many healthcare providers, CAM use by patients presents a professional challenge. CAM therapies are not routinely included in nursing and medical school curricula. As a result, many clinicians are not comfortable with their level of expertise with wide-ranging CAM therapies or with discussing CAM use by patients. Other practitioners may fear they have personal biases and judgments that threaten an open dialogue with patients concerning CAM. Many HCPs possess a traditional background with little or no knowledge of data related to the efficacy and safety of CAM therapies and harbor skepticism related to safety, efficacy, and cost—resulting in hesitancy to include it as part of the plan of care.

Most physicians did not routinely discuss CAM therapies with their patients even when aware that these products and practices may interact with conventional therapies in helpful or harmful ways (Angell & Kassirer, 1998; Eisenberg et al., 1993; Eisenberg, 1997; Ernst & Cassileth, 1998). Wynia et al. (1999) found, "Physicians were more likely to discuss CAM therapies with patients they knew or suspected to be using them, but even during visits with these patients fewer than half (44%) would discuss CAM therapies" (p. 451). Only one quarter of the physicians surveyed discussed the use of CAM therapies with most new HIV-infected patients, and only 5% discussed these therapies at most follow-up visits with these patients. Even fewer regularly discussed CAM therapies with non-HIV-infected patients. This was surprising because more than one third (36%) of the HCPs responding reported using CAM therapies themselves, and the majority (63%) thought CAM therapies were often or usually helpful for this patient population.

There are few studies on nurses' response to CAM use by patients (Fitch, Gray, Greenberg, Lebrecque & Douglas, 1999; Oncology Nursing Society, n.d.; Salmenpera, Suominen, & Lauri, 1998). Wang & Yates (2006) conducted a grounded theory study where associated themes related to the core category, Being Responsive, reflected findings of previous studies. In some instances, nurses openly supported the use of CAMs and acknowledged the benefits while advising continued investigation of benefits and risks. Others were skeptical, "most acknowledging they would not interfere with patients' final decisions" (p. 290). Some nurses were ambivalent as long as the interventions were not harmful. However, they stressed the need for the development of an evidence base in support of CAMs and the importance of continuing discussion of all interventions and products used by patients in their practices.

RESPONSIBILITIES OF HEALTHCARE PROVIDERS

One physician stated, "I'm damned if I do and damned if I don't." Asking about CAM use left the HCP open to the need to evaluate and respond to CAM use by patients. This would involve lengthier visits and/or more coordination with team members or certified CAM practitioners. Not asking, though, would be an ethical and legal risk if patients' health care or treatment were compromised by undisclosed use of CAM therapies. Weigner et al. (2002, p. 889) proposed evaluating CAMs used or considered by patients along a continuum that ranges from "recommend" to "accept" to "discourage."

But how to begin a patient care session where discussion of CAM therapies should be as routine as taking vital signs or asking about conventional medications and treatments? Each practitioner needs to look inward and honestly examine both visceral responses to and scientific knowledge of CAM therapies. Personal philosophy along with experience and knowledge of CAMs may influence discussions between practitioner and patient about CAM use. Both comfort and knowledge are the foundations for therapeutic and beneficial discussion of CAM with patients.

The HCP does not need to approve CAM use by patients, but does need to present sound advice based on scientific evidence to integrate CAM preferences of patients while minimizing possible risks and interactions. NCCAM reports on clinical trials that have looked at efficacy, end points, and side effects of CAM use and provides a compilation of results from systematic reviews and meta-analyses. Specific disease processes, symptoms, and quality-of-life concerns are presented with the benefits and risks of select CAM products and practices. Referral to a practitioner competent and credentialed in the CAM-specific area is also an option for HCPs who are not comfortable discussing complementary and alternative therapy use by patients in their practices.

Inpatient and outpatient practice areas should develop protocols for the CAM therapies most frequently utilized by the patient population served. These guidelines, developed from evidence-based reports, can be used to initiate discussions as well as direct care decisions. HCPs can seek personal continuing education opportunities in CAM and request presentations by expert CAM practitioners targeted for practitioners, patients, and the public.

HCPs can encourage their respective professional educational institutions to add substantial information and discussion of CAM therapies to curricula. Wetzel, Kaptchuk, Haramati, and Eisenberg (2003) discuss integration into medical education curricula and course objectives. The principles of biofeedback and stress reduction can be integrated into physiology classes. Discussions of dietary interventions and supplements may be woven into nutrition classes while herbal remedies are addressed in relation to specific disease entities. Each professional group represented on the healthcare team can be encouraged to include CAM therapies, when appropriate, during rounds, team meetings, and case study presentations, and in so doing, present an integrative rather than complementary/alternative approach to care.

The success of discussions between healthcare providers and patients is anchored in the basic principles of therapeutic communication. The essential intervention is to listen with an open mind and explore the patient's hopes and fears in relation to the disease, treatment, and effects on their life. Fletcher, as cited in Marshall (2001), encourages practitioners to recognize their own personal values that may interfere with effective client communication; to explore client fears, hopes, and wishes; and to be empathic when supplying objective information. Scientific objectivity and support can then be balanced.

CAM RESOURCES

There are an increasing number of peer-reviewed studies of CAM therapies. The Cochrane Library is a collection of databases that contain high-quality, independent evidence to inform healthcare decision making. Cochrane Reviews represent the highest level of evidence on which to base clinical treatment decisions. In addition to Cochrane Reviews, "the Cochrane Library provides other sources of reliable information: other systematic reviews abstracts, technology assessments, economic evaluations, and individual clinical trials—all the current evidence in one single environment" (Cochran Reviews, n.d.). NCCAM publishes fact sheets that can be used to provide information on CAM for HCPs and patients and can also be used to initiate CAM conversations. These fact sheets include basic information on the selected product or service and a summary of research in both professional and lay terms. Reviews of specific products and services, such as acupuncture, provide information on their effects on disease progression and survival, symptom relief, contraindications, adverse effects, and interactions with other CAM therapies and conventional treatment.

Weigner et al. (2002) conducted a comprehensive review of the safety and efficacy of several CAM therapies in an attempt to summarize current evidence. The depth and strength of this evidence varies widely by CAM therapy, some being studied more rigorously and extensively. Scholarly studies from major professional journals and submissions from CAM-related databases were reviewed. Also included in the review were several Web sites, including the National Cancer Institute, the Center for Alternative Medicine Research in Cancer at the University of Texas at Houston Health Sciences Center, and the American Cancer Society. These sites provide publications and links that can be helpful to the reader seeking rigorous clinical trial results of CAM therapies as well as anecdotal and observational reports.

"The Natural Medicines Comprehensive Database (NMCD) is a resource for information on herbs, dietary supplements, alternative systems of medicine, vitamin and mineral ingredients of currently available natural medicines. The practitioner or consumer can locate reliable information on herbal remedies, dietary supplements, vitamins, minerals, and other natural products and their targeted use. In addition, safety and effectiveness ratings for each product can be found by using the Natural Product/Drug Interaction Checker to test for harmful interactions. This Consumer version of Natural Medicines Comprehensive Database provides easy-to-understand information" (M. D. Anderson Cancer Center, n.d.).

MOVING FORWARD

HCPs and patients are encouraged to reflect on the knowledge, skills, and attitudes needed to make care decisions about CAM therapies. It is not necessary, or even realistic, to know everything about all CAM therapies. It is helpful, however, to be aware of clinical trials on CAM therapies being conducted at major academic and medical institutions and the National Institutes of Health. A visit to the NCCAM Web site will reveal an updated list of major CAM therapies and scholarly information for both professionals and nonprofessionals interested in CAM. In an innovative approach, the Center for Mind-Body Medicine in Washington, DC, has created a program to train "integrative-care counselors." The trained counselors then provide patients with practical assistance in assessing and choosing CAM therapies and creating individualized programs of comprehensive care that are individualized as well as safe (http://www.cmbm.org).

However, the use of resources alone, without open discussion between caregivers and patients, is valueless. What is necessary for complete and holistic care is communication: patient to HCP, HCP to patient, and HCPs among themselves. One way to initiate a discussion about CAM use is to ask, "Tell me how you have been feeling. What have you found helpful when you feel this way?" Questions related to the use of CAMs also can be seamlessly integrated into discussions of lifestyle, diet, or medication review. Correa-Velez et al. (2005, p. 954) posed a question in their qualitative study that could serve as an excellent discussion opener: "Could you tell me more about your past experiences using complementary and alternative medicine?"

Another way to open a discussion on present and past use of CAM is to simply add specific CAM questions on the patient health assessment form. A patient can also be asked to keep a record or diary of everything they eat, inhale, inject, apply, bring home from the general food market or health food store, and get from friends or other sources. One place for the patient to easily record this information is on a cell phone note pad or other personal electronic device. This record is an excellent way to approach the topic of CAM use and can be very revealing.

HCPs must balance evidence-based advice with respect for patients who seek survival benefits, relief of symptoms, or improved well-being or quality of life. During discussions with patients, each practitioner should be mindful of nonverbal behavior: Am I frowning, shaking my head, or looking away? What about language used: Does my choice of words convey disapproval? Am I assessing, discussing, or reprimanding? Gordon (2001, p. 47) refers to HCPs as "healing partners" to help choose therapies, both mainstream and CAM, that best meet individual needs. As a partner, each HCP should listen nonjudgmentally and present CAM options within safe parameters while supporting the patient in his or her decisions.

Wetzel et al. (2003, p. 193) so perfectly state, "There should be room for healthy diversity and pluralism of ideas, with respectful coordination, integration, and opportunity for acceptance or rejection." Evidence-based practice is not only the results of clinical trials, but also those results combined with professional expertise and individual client situation and preferences. If CAM therapies are what the patient seeks, the practitioner can offer those that are safe and appear to meet patient goals. Close follow-up is necessary, however, to assess for adverse effects or interference with conventional therapies. NCCAM also refers to the use of CAM as complementary/integrative medicine. This can be seen as a description that marries traditional and complementary approaches rather than continuing the assumption that CAM is outside the range of possible treatment options.

CONCLUSION

HCP acceptance of the use of CAM therapies is not a blanket endorsement, but rather a realization that patients may have different definitions of benefit and harm. The ultimate goal is to locate the balance between individual patient autonomy and evidence-based practice. Perhaps the real question for the HCP is not "if" to honor patients' choices to use CAM therapies, but rather "when, where, and how," while remaining comfortable with professional ethical values and concerns.

This article briefly touches on the multitude of CAM therapies possible and some of the concerns of both HCPs and patients. My wish is that the information presented here will serve as a guide to weighing the benefits of the full spectrum of healing interventions that are compatible with the goals of both the person with cancer and professional care partners.

Lynda Shand, PhD, received her BSN from Seton Hall University in 1973. She began her nursing career in the Pediatric Division of United Hospitals of Newark, NJ. An MA in nursing education in 1981 from New York University allowed her to combine her interests in pediatric nursing and teaching in many diverse settings. Dr. Shand completed her PhD at New York University in 1998 while working as a clinical research nurse affiliated with the National Institutes of Health in the areas of Maternal-Child HIV/AIDS and Adult Oncology. She participated in the End-of-Life Nursing Education Consortium (ELNEC) and is certified to provide the ELNEC education modules to healthcare professionals. ELNEC is a national education program to improve care provided by nurses to patients and their families facing the complexities of life-threatening illness and is funded by a grant from the Robert Wood Johnson Foundation. Her areas of teaching as an associate professor at the College of New Rochelle include pediatrics, nursing education, and palliative/hospice care.

REFERENCES

Adler, S. R., & Fosket, J. R. (1999). Disclosing complementary and alternative medicine use in the medical encounter: A qualitative study in women with breast cancer. *Journal of Family Practice, 48,* 453–458.

American Cancer Society. (n.d.). *Statistics for 2008.* Retrieved July 23, 2009, from http://www.cancer.org/docroot/STT/stt_0_2008.asp?sitearea=Stt&level=1

Angell, M., & Kassirer, J. (1998). Alternative medicine: the risks of untested and unregulated remedies. *New England Journal of Medicine, 339*(12), 839–841.

Austin, J. A. (1998). Why patients use alternative medicine: Results of a national study. *JAMA, 279,* 1548–1553.

Barnes, P. M., Powell-Griner, E., McFann, K., & Nahin, R. L. (2004). Complementary and alternative medicine use among adults: United States, 2002. *Advance Data, 343,* 1–19.

Cassileth, B. R., Schraub, S., Robinson, E., & Vickers, A. (2001). Alternative medicine use worldwide: The international union against cancer survey. *Cancer, 91,* 1390–1393.

Center for Mind-Body Medicine. (n.d.). Retrieved July 23, 2009, from http://www.cmbm.org.

Chatwin, J., & Tovey, P. (2004). Complementary and alternative medicine (CAM), cancer and group-based actions: A critical review of the literature. *European Journal of Cancer Care, 13*(3), 210–218.

Cochrane Reviews. (n.d.). Product Descriptions. Retrieved July 23, 2009, from http://www3.interscience.wiley.com/cgi-bin/mrwhome/106568753/ProductDescriptions.html

Correa-Velez, I., Clavino, A., & Eastwood, H. (2005). Surviving, relieving, repairing, and boosting up: Reasons for using complementary/alternative medicine among patients with advanced cancer: A thematic analysis. *Journal of Palliative Medicine, 8*(5), 953–961.

Coss, R. A., McGrath, P., & Caggiano, V. (1998). Alternative care: Patient choices for adjunct therapies within a cancer center. *Cancer Practice, 6*(3), 176–181.

Eisenberg, D. M. (1997). Advising patients who seek alternative medical therapies. *Annals of Internal Medicine, 127,* 61–69.

Eisenberg, D. M., Ettner, S. L., Appel, S., Wilkey, S., VanRompay, M., & Kessler, R. (1998). Trends in alternative medicine use in the United States, 1990-1997: Results of a follow-up national survey. *JAMA, 280*(18), 1569–1575.

Eisenberg, D. M., Kessler, R. C., Foster, C., Norlock, F. E., Calkins, D. R., & Delbanco, T. (1993). Unconventional medicine in the United States: Prevalence, costs, and patterns of use. *New England Journal of Medicine, 328*(4), 246–252.

Elliot, J., Kealey, C., & Oliver, I. (2008). (Using) complementary and alternative medicine: The perceptions of palliative patients with cancer. *Journal of Palliative Medicine, 11*(1), 58–67.

Ernst, E., & Cassileth, B. R. (1998). The prevalence of complementary medicine in cancer: A systematic review. *Cancer, 83,* 777–782.

Evans, M. A., Shaw, A. R., Sharp, D. J., Thompson, E. A., Falk, E., Turton, P., et al. (2007). Men with cancer: Is their use of complementary and alternative medicine a response to unmet needs by conventional care? *European Journal of Cancer Care, 16*(6), 517–525.

Fitch, M., Gray, R., Greenberg, M., Lebrecque, M., & Douglas, M. (1999). Nurses' perspectives on unconventional therapies. *Cancer Nursing, 22*(3), 238–245.

Fouladbakhsh, J., Stommel, M., Given, B., & Given, C. (2005). Predictors of use of complementary and alternative therapies among patients with cancer. *Oncology Nursing Forum, 32*(6), 1115–1122.

Gordon, J. (2001). Creating comprehensive cancer care. *Cancer Practice, 9*(1), 47–49.

Gray, R., Fitch, M., Greenberg, M., Voros, P., Douglas, M., & Lebrecque, M. (1997). Physicians' perspectives on unconventional therapies. *Journal of Palliative Care, 13,* 14–21.

Humpel, N. (2006). Gaining insight into what, why and where of complementary and alternative medicine use by cancer patients and survivors. *European Journal of Cancer Care, 15*(4), 362–368.

Jordan, M., & Delunas, L. (2001). Quality of life and patterns of non-traditional therapy used by patients with cancer. *Oncology Nursing Forum*, *28*(7), 1107–1113.

M. D. Anderson Cancer Center. (n.d.). Retrieved July 20, 2009, from http://www.mdanderson.org/education-and-research/resources-for-professionals/clinical-tools-and-resources/cimer/index.html

Mao, J., Farrar, J., Xie, S., Bowman, M., & Armstrong, K. (2007). Use of complementary and alternative medicine and prayer among a national sample of cancer survivors when compared to other populations without cancer. *Complementary Therapies in Medicine*, *15*(1), 21–29.

Marshall, P. (2001). Alternative and complementary therapies among cancer patients: Nursing considerations. *Kansas Nurse*, *76*(3), 1, 3–8.

Michaud, L. (2000). BCOP complementary/alternative therapies: Potential safety issues in cancer care. *Cancer Practice*, *8*, 243–247.

Molassiotis, A., Fernandez-Ortega, P., Pud, D., Ozden, G., Scott, G., Panteli, V., et al. (2005). Use of complementary and alternative medicine in cancer patients: A European survey. *Annals of Oncology*, *16*(4), 655–663.

National Center for Complementary and Alternative Medicine. (n.d.). Retrieved July 20, 2009, from http://nccam.nih.gov/health/whatiscam/overview.htm

National Center for Complementary and Alternative Medicine. (n.d.). Retrieved July 20, 2009, from http://nccam.nih.gov/timetotalk/backgrounder.htm

National Center for Complementary and Alternative Medicine. (n.d.). Retrieved July 20, 2009, from http://nccam.nih.gov/health/acupuncture/acupuncture-for-pain.htm

National Institutes of Health. (1998). NIH Consensus Conference. Acupuncture. *The Journal of the American Medical Association*, *280*(17), 1518–1524.

Natural Medicines Comprehensive Database. (n.d.). Retrieved July 23, 2009, from http://www.mdanderson.org/education-and-research/resources-for-professionals/clinical-tools-and-resources/cimer/therapies/index.html

Oncology Nursing Society. (n.d). The use of complementary, alternative, and integrative therapies in cancer care. Retrieved on July 22, 2009, from http://www.ons.org/Publications/Positions/ComplementaryTherapies.shtml

Ott, M. (2002). Complementary and alternative therapies in cancer symptom management. *Cancer Practice, 10*(3), 162–166.

Peace, G., & Manesse, A. (2002). The Cavendish Centre for integrated cancer care: Assessment of patient needs and responses. *Complementary Therapy in Medicine, 10*(1), 33–41.

Salmenpera, L., Suominen, T., & Lauri, S. (1998). Oncology nurses' attitudes towards alternative medicine. *Psycho-Oncology, 7*(6), 449–453.

Sloman, R., Brown, P., Aldana, E., & Chee, E. (1994). The use of relaxation for the promotion of comfort and pain relief in persons with advanced cancer. *Contemp Nurse, 3*, 6–12.

Sollner, W., Maislinger, S., DeVries, A., Steixner, E., Rumpold, G., & Lukas, P. (2000). Use of complementary and alternative medicine by cancer patients is not associated with perceived distress or poor compliance with standard treatment but with active coping behavior. *Cancer, 89*(4), 873–880.

Sparber, A., Bauer, L., Curt, G., Eisenberg, D., Levin, T., Parks, S., et al. (2000). Use of complementary medicine by adult patients participating in cancer clinical trials. *Oncology Nursing Forum, 27*(4), 623–630.

Syrjala, K., Donaldson, G., Davis, M., Kippes, M., & Carr, J. (1995). Relaxation and imagery and cognitive behavioral training reduce pain during cancer treatment: A controlled clinical trial. *Pain, 63*, 189–198.

Tasaki, K., Maskarinec, G., Shumay, D., Tatsumura, Y., & Kakai, Y. (2002). Communication between physicians and cancer patients about complementary and alternative medicine: Exploring patients' perspectives. *Psycho-Oncology, 11*, 212–220.

Wang, S., & Yates, P. (2006). Nurses' responses to people with cancer who use complementary and alternative medicine. *International Journal of Nursing Practice, 12*, 288–294.

Weigner, W., Smith, M., Boon, H., Richardson, M., Kaptchuk, T., & Eisenberg, D. (2002). Advising patients who seek complementary and alternative therapies for cancer. *Annals of Internal Medicine, 137*(11), 889–913.

Wetzel, M., Kaptchuk, T., Haramati, A., & Eisenberg, D. (2003). Complementary and alternative medical therapies: Implications for medical intervention. *Annals of Internal Medicine, 138*(3), 191–196.

Wiley Interscience. The Cochrane Library. Accessed July 21, 2009, from http://www3.interscience.wiley.com/cgi-bin/mrwhome/106568753/ ProductDescriptions.html

Wynia, M., Eisenberg, D., & Wilson, I. (1999). Physician-patient communication about complementary and alternative medical therapies: A survey of physicians caring for patients with human immunodeficiency virus infection. *The Journal of Alternative and Complementary Medicine, 5,* 447–456.

CHAPTER 7

Ethical Dilemmas in the Treatment of Cancer

Nancy Berlinger and Bruce Jennings

E thical dilemmas arise from medicine's incomplete power and mixed blessings. This may be more evident in oncology than in any other field. When cancer can be cured, few ethical issues arise. When "management" or "control" rather than cure is the goal, or when the prospects of cure are highly uncertain, many issues arise. When cancer treatment becomes chronic disease management, discussing and making decisions about treatment may be medically complex for patients, families, and clinicians alike. These decisions are also ethically (intellectually, emotionally, and relationally) complex, due to the personal and family issues at stake, as well as the uncertainty of prognosis and of treatment's impact on quality of life. New treatment options and new ways of thinking about the goals of cancer treatment also add to the difficulty of these decisions. Newer therapies may offer uncertain or marginal benefit and significant toxicity. Then there is the growing recognition that the burdens of attempting to treat advanced cancer are likely to be financial as well as physiological; the extremely high cost of some newer cancer treatments further complicates decision making.

What counts as a benefit? What should be done when further treatment is no longer worth its physiological or financial cost? These questions have ethical, research, and policy dimensions, but they must be addressed within the physician-patient relationship in the treatment of advanced cancer (Fojo & Grady, 2009). In this chapter we review the changing landscape of cancer treatment and its ethical challenges for oncologists and other cancer treatment specialists, palliative care specialists, and hospice professionals, as well as for patients and families.

MANAGING CANCER AS A CHRONIC DISEASE

Over the past two decades, the landscape for cancer patients diagnosed with primary or recurrent advanced (Stages III or IV) disease has shifted significantly. At one time the cancer treatment process for such patients usually involved a drastic, but short-term effort to slow the progression of the disease, followed by a dying experience marked, if the patient was fortunate, by good symptom management and holistic hospice or palliative care. Now the course of cancer treatment, even in advanced stages, may be longer and the boundary less distinct between disease-modifying treatment and pain and symptom management. Today some cancers that cannot be cured can be stabilized and managed as chronic diseases. The number of chemotherapy options continues to grow, as do other treatment options for ameliorating certain types of advanced cancer. These options include biologic therapies that aim to interfere with the growth of cancer cells. The treatment of metastatic breast cancer, in particular, now potentially includes many different therapies, although the options that may benefit a particular patient depend on this patient's treatment history, hormone receptor status, and individual responsiveness to specific agents (Hillner & Smith, 2009). The standard approach to treating chronic myelogenous leukemia has been significantly changed by the introduction of an effective long-term oral therapy that targets enzymes involved in cancer cell growth.

The emergence of oral chemotherapies illustrates how the natural history of some cancers is being affected by a chronic-disease approach emphasizing control rather than cure, and how this gradual shift is affecting the lived experience of some persons with common types of cancer. A report from the National Comprehensive Cancer Network (2008) described the advent of oral chemotherapy (a term that may include orally administered biologic agents as well as cytotoxic agents) as a development that "will significantly impact all aspects of oncology care." It is already shifting certain responsibilities from professionals to patients themselves, as is typical in a chronic-disease paradigm. Oral chemotherapy is "real" chemotherapy. While some patients may find daily oral regimens easier to tolerate than weekly IV therapy, and while oral chemotherapy prescriptions are filled at a pharmacy, these regimens can be burdensome and their side effects significant. This shift also has social consequences. For patients with advanced disease, using IV chemotherapy may be a familiar ritual: Patients may even try to book their appointments around the schedule of a favorite nurse who offers encouragement. Oral chemotherapy is more private and less time consuming, but it is also more isolating. It requires patients to keep track of dosages and side effects, to maintain contact with clinicians by phone or e-mail rather than in person, and to obtain psychological support outside of the structure provided by the chemotherapy suite and related clinical appointments. The rituals of outpatient cancer treatment have not yet adapted to this new treatment modality. Finally, the shift has economic consequences. As oral chemotherapies tend to be expensive, patients' ability to benefit from them may be constrained by their prescription drug coverage. Researchers have documented cost as one of the reasons patients may not adhere to oral regimens. Worry about the cost of treatment adds to treatment burden.

Moreover, while some oral chemotherapies may be effective long-term therapies for some patients, other patients may obtain more limited benefits and will eventually need to begin or return to IV chemotherapy. A clinician may not make a sharp distinction between an orally administered agent and an intravenously administered agent in terms of effectiveness. These regimens may hold different meanings for patients, for whom a shift from oral to IV chemotherapy may symbolize progression in a way that other changes in treatment do not.

As these developments suggest, the concept of chronicity is still emerging in cancer treatment. Oncologists may use the term "chronic" in conversations with patients, to characterize disease that is not curable, but is stable or in the process of being stabilized in response to treatment. Due to the availability of a wider range of potentially effective therapies, some oncologists already characterize advanced breast cancer as a chronic disease (Dufresne et al., 2008). As noted, some forms of leukemia and lymphoma may also be treated and managed as chronic diseases. However, if some forms of cancer are—or are slowly becoming—chronic diseases, they are unlike many other conditions that individuals learn to live and cope with over a long period of time. Most cancer treatments, as well as public perceptions of how cancer treatments work, are still organized around "cure." The stigma and psychological burden of living with a life-threatening chronic disease may therefore be greater when that disease is cancer.

However, oncology professionals have not yet agreed on an ethical framework for managing cancer as a chronic disease. There is an established paradigm for primary-care clinicians treating patients with chronic disease (Bodenheimer, Lorig, Holman, & Grumbach, 2002). However, this paradigm, grounded in shared decision making and in support for patient self-management, was not developed within the specialized context of cancer treatment. Hospice and palliative care were developed with reference to the needs of cancer patients and their families and are based on a shared decision-making paradigm, but they were not conceptualized as chronic-disease services. Indeed, the social mandate of hospice, as symbolized in the 6-month prognosis criterion of the Medicare hospice benefit, has been just the opposite: The shortest good-byes are best. We know that this is not true.

Cancer is also different from other common life-threatening diseases that can be managed as chronic diseases through long-term adherence to an established treatment regimen, such as dialysis for end-stage renal disease, insulin injections for diabetes, or antiretroviral drugs for HIV/AIDS. As cancer tends to become resistant to a particular therapy, long-term management of the disease often requires frequent changes in treatment regimens. Each new drug may bring new side effects and may require new supplemental treatments that add their own burdens. The psychological burden of living with the disease that will probably kill you is compounded by uncertainty over whether your current regimen is working, or if it will be replaced by a different regimen that you must learn and adapt to, physically and psychologically. One of the goals of chronic care is to find a mode of accommodation to treatment and the limitations imposed by impairment that is compatible with a meaningful self-identity and mode of life (Jennings, Caplan, & Callahan, 1988). However, cancer is notoriously subversive of a comfortable, stable modus vivendi.

CANCER SURVIVORSHIP AS IDENTITY, GOAL, AND CHALLENGE

The idea of "surviving" cancer adds another layer of complexity to cancer treatment. Federal agencies that track cancer statistics define a cancer survivor as a person living with a prior diagnosis of cancer. However, a cancer center's institutional definition of survivorship may be more narrow, focusing on services for patients who have completed treatment and are dealing with posttreatment needs, such as counseling or rehabilitative therapy. Media and marketing depictions of cancer survivors—think of advertisements aimed at prospective patients for cancer centers—focus on stories about being cured of cancer, not about being treated continuously for a chronic disease. Becoming a survivor may be a clinical goal and a personal identity for some patients. Even after patients recognize that they have a form of cancer that cannot be cured— that they will never be "posttreatment"—they must rely on some available language of self-description. Even if some of these patients do not self-identify as "survivors," they may have no alternative but to rely on language suggesting that cure is still a possibility, that they'll "beat this thing" someday. Families, friends, and acquaintances also rely on this way of thinking and talking. So do clinicians, who often characterize a decision to continue chemotherapy as continuing to "fight," and may refer to highly toxic—but not necessarily highly effective—therapies using a battlefield analogy: "the big guns." If this battle cannot be won, if these weapons are likely to inflict more damage on the patient than on the target, these metaphors may undermine the process of informed consent, by suggesting that burdens represent benefits. Chronicity in cancer needs its own narrative and its own metaphors. It does not have them yet.

The idea, or ideal, of cancer survivorship has ethical implications, because it may influence treatment decision making near the end of life. Cancer patients who have used different therapies, in some cases over years, to prevent or treat recurrences or to keep advanced disease stable have made many decisions in favor of continuing treatment, and continuing to live with cancer. It is therefore profoundly difficult for them, or for their families, to consider the option of forgoing treatment. This is clear from extensive studies that conclude that patients who are near the end of life will still continue to pursue treatment. It is part of the same syndrome that leads to the underutilization of palliative care, if palliative care is associated with "giving up," and to very late referrals to hospice programs. Given the "fighting" metaphors that pervade cancer treatment, forgoing treatment may feel like surrendering: a failure of courage, a moral wrong.

THE ROLE OF CLINICAL TRIALS AND NOVEL THERAPIES

The option of clinical trials also complicates decisions about withholding and withdrawing cancer treatment near the end of life. Patients and caregivers can obtain information about clinical trials from public databases such as the National Cancer Institute's clinical trial registry. For some cancers, there may be hundreds of active trials underway at any one time. Some research participants obtain therapeutic benefits from experimental drugs, although such benefits are incidental to the goals of clinical research. Others may recognize that they are participating in research and realize that this is research precisely because the benefits are unknown, but still hope for individual benefit. These research participants are able to know and to hope at the same time. Unfortunately, some patients may not understand the distinction between participation in a research protocol and receiving individualized therapy; this is called the "therapeutic misconception" by ethicists (Appelbaum, Roth, Lidz, Benson, & Winslade, 1987). Media coverage of promising (or hyped) drugs in the research pipeline contributes to popular beliefs that experimental (or newer or more expensive) drugs are better drugs. This may lead to the mischaracterization of a highly experimental therapy or a Phase I toxicity trial as a "last shot" or a "miracle drug" by patients or families who want—or demand—to be "doing something." Clinicians sometimes comply with these wishes or demands without clarifying how the burdens and risks of trial participation differ from the benefits and burdens of treatment.

The therapeutic misconception is a clear-cut ethical problem in medicine. "The dying cancer patient in a Phase I trial" may even function as shorthand for it. However, the relationship between treatment and research in cancer care is more complex than this term suggests. Among cancer patients with advanced disease, there may be no bright line between treatment and research, particularly at academic medical centers and in pediatric oncology. Oncologists, patients, and family caregivers may discuss treatment options that include long-established regimens; newly approved therapies; and clinical trials that may include combinations of approved drugs, or of approved drugs and experimental therapies. More controversial are treatments that involve (a) the off-label use of therapies that have been approved for a specific cancer or patient population before these therapies have gone through wider-use studies to determine whether they are safe and effective treatments for other cancers or populations; and (b) the individualized, off-protocol use of still-experimental therapies.

THE KEY ETHICAL ISSUE: WEIGHING BENEFITS AND BURDENS

In many domains of critical and terminal care, the hardest ethical issues are those that arise in situations where the patient has lost decision-making capacity and the surrogate must make treatment decisions guided by what is known about the patient's values and preferences. Cancer is a life-threatening condition that may not compromise the patient's decision-making capacity until very near death, when there may be no more decisions left to make. As such, the ethical principle of autonomy, exercised through the actions of giving informed consent or informed refusal, provides straightforward theoretical guidance.

However, as we have seen, it is no easier for the patient to make decisions—in particular, to decide to forgo further treatment—than for a loved one or another designated surrogate to decide. Society may be more comfortable when the patient decides to forgo further treatment than when a surrogate makes this decision, but that does not mean that the patient's autonomous decision is not psychologically difficult and fraught with ethical challenges. An autonomous person has a right to choose, but how should he exercise that right? What responsibilities does a person have to herself and to others? These are ethical questions, and this is where the weighing of benefits and burdens comes in.

Like much else in cancer care, benefits and burdens are entangled, and thinking them through is a complex task. It should never be presumed that research participants who reasonably hope for therapeutic benefit are automatically falling prey to the therapeutic misconception. However, if therapeutic misconception is present, it will be difficult for a patient to weigh benefits and burdens because this patient's conceptual understanding of treatment is flawed: By definition, this patient believes, incorrectly, that the burdens and risks of participating in a clinical trial will yield individualized therapeutic benefits. Even if therapeutic misconception is not present, or if cancer treatment is taking place outside of a research institution, cancer patients are likely to be aware of and affected by the continuous introduction of new therapies—some of which reflect true scientific innovations, others of which build on existing knowledge. In the field of oncology, many have expressed concern over the routine characterization of novel therapies as breakthroughs and the rapid adoption of these therapies as standard treatment (Fojo & Grady, 2009, p. 1). Manufacturers justify the extremely high prices of these new drugs by touting their life-saving benefits, even though these drugs may have provided only marginal benefit to trial participants while adding significant burdens through toxicity. Suppose a drug offers little or no possibility of prolonging overall survival. Or suppose it offers, at best, a progression-free survival measured in days or weeks, during which a patient may become sicker due to toxic side effects. Should this drug be presented as a valid treatment option?

On the other hand, should oncologists avoid recommending certain drugs until there is solid evidence that benefits will exceed burdens? It is difficult to be opposed to evidence-based medicine. However, this approach, which is conservative in the face of uncertainty and makes sense when applied to populations, may not make sense to individual patients. A strict evidence-based approach may not make sense to oncologists, either, as they have observed that the treatments that do work do so before they have been proven to work. The clinical trial process does not make a drug effective, but aims to distinguish safe and effective drugs from unsafe and ineffective drugs, and to understand a potential treatment's benefits and burdens. What do we say to those patients who could have benefited during the gap between hypothesis and confirmation, but were denied access to a still-experimental drug?

And what about cost and access? Do oncologists have an obligation to inform patients and families that a new drug of uncertain benefit will cost thousands of dollars per month? Do professional and advocacy groups in cancer care have an obligation to confront pharmaceutical manufacturers about the practice of setting an extremely high price on resources that are—or are promoted as—life saving, a state of affairs that some oncologists themselves have begun to call "profiteering"? (Hillner & Smith, 2009, p. 2112) Even if prices were controlled or subsidized, many cancer therapies would still be out of the reach of the uninsured and would still exceed the lifetime limits of many patients with health insurance. These urgent questions have implications for communications among oncologists, patients, and family caregivers whenever a treatment regimen stops working and the possibility of a new drug, of uncertain benefit and certain burden, is introduced.

CANCER TREATMENT AND HOSPICE CARE—OPEN ACCESS
Hospice programs trace their roots to the care of patients dying of cancer, and hospice continues to be closely—but no longer exclusively—identified with the care of cancer patients following a decision to forgo further therapeutic treatment. In 2007, cancer patients made up approximately 41% of those enrolled in hospice nationwide (National Hospice and Palliative Care Organization, 2008). However, in the American hospice community, an "open-access" movement now permits hospice-eligible patients to continue to receive some therapeutic treatments aimed at symptom control while receiving optimal palliative care and other services, such as nursing care, under the Medicare hospice benefit (Abelson, 2007). Some hospices can now accept patients who are receiving life-prolonging and disease-modifying cancer treatment that is covered by another insurer. This emerging approach does not place an unsustainable financial burden on hospice programs, as some expensive high-tech palliative measures have threatened to do in the past. These changes in hospice reflect efforts to help more patients who may be near the end of life to benefit from hospice services for longer periods. They also reflect continuing changes in what cancer treatment is, what it means to patients, how it is delivered, and how oncologists and patients manage advanced disease and its impact on a patient's overall health and life.

Nonetheless, open access raises other ethical questions. Can and should hospice programs accommodate and subsidize the care of individual patients who want to continue to receive therapeutic treatment but do not have insurance to cover the cost of these treatments? For open-access patients, the nursing and other care and support they need may be more intense than it is with traditional hospice patients. Is this an equitable distribution of resources within a hospice program? Will open access be constrained by the financial resources of individual hospice programs and be unavailable to patients served by smaller programs? Is it a sustainable model for hospice in the long term?

A further issue involves the question of which treatments may be incompatible with hospice care. For example, certain interventions, such as video-assisted thorascopic surgery (VATS) to relieve pain and dyspnea caused by large pleural effusions, are palliative in intent and surgical in nature, and require hospitalization. Such interventions may be undertaken to relieve pain and symptoms and also to facilitate the continuation of chemotherapy, radiation, or other potentially life-prolonging treatment. Combining these interventions with hospice will require new approaches to collaboration among hospice providers and oncologists, surgeons, and other professionals who may continue to be involved in the care of patients under an open-access model.

Whether or not a patient is enrolled in open-access hospice, professionals responsible for interventions that seek to relieve pain or symptoms (such as the thoracic surgeon who performs the VATS procedure) should recognize that they, too, are palliative care providers, and should seek to collaborate with palliative care specialists on the care of individual patients. If an institution's structure works against collaboration, or if professional training in palliative medicine fails to reach specialists who may be involved in pain and symptom management but do not self-identify as palliative care providers, these structural flaws have ethical consequences.

DISCUSSING THE GOALS OF CANCER TREATMENT WITHIN THE GOALS OF CARE

Benefits and burdens are difficult to assess in the abstract; they need to be anchored in particular goals. When a patient is diagnosed with metastatic (Stage IV) disease, or experiences metastatic progression or a metastatic recurrence, the oncologist should clarify the goals of treatment when disease cannot be cured. These goals—which may include preventing disease progression, relieving pain or other symptoms, improving functioning, and prolonging life—should be referred to as treatment continues, modified if necessary as the disease progresses, and shared with other professionals involved in the patient's care. Goal setting and treatment planning create a framework for discussing the benefits and burdens of any particular regimen (Harrington

& Smith, 2008). Clarifying the goals of treatment is also important when a patient is diagnosed with a form of cancer that is treatable but likely to recur.

The oncologist should also find out how a patient prefers to receive information about treatment and prognosis in between more structured deliberations about treatment decisions. Some patients prefer to be kept up to date continuously. Others prefer to ask the oncologist specific questions as they arise. Still others prefer to involve a surrogate or other caregiver in receiving information and in maintaining communications with professionals. As a patient's preferences concerning the flow of information may change over the course of treatment, and as some patients may be unsure about how to open a conversation, some oncologists give patients diagnosed with advanced disease a list of sample questions to establish open communications and to signal, you can ask me anything, anytime (Glynne-Jones et al., 2006; Harrington & Smith, 2008).

The goals of cancer treatment are not the same as a patient's own goals of care, which may include their reasons for pursuing or continuing treatment as well as the aspects of treatment they wish to avoid. The goals of a patient who has young children are likely to include both "staying alive for my children" and "avoiding treatments that disrupt my family's life." This patient's first goal may be obvious to her oncologist; the second goal may be less obvious and is likely to exist in tension with the first goal. Establishing and documenting the patient's goals of care through a formal process of advance care planning, before a seriously ill patient faces a decision about a particular treatment, may create a useful framework for bringing the patient's values and preferences concerning quality of life into ongoing conversations and decisions about treatment. This framework may be especially helpful when a particular treatment offers little chance of adding to quantity of life. If patient, family, and professional have been talking about quality of life over months or years of treatment, they may be better prepared to assess a potential new treatment in terms of its qualitative benefits and burdens. Some treatments create burdens that are not physiological. The location, frequency, and other requirements of various treatment options, including scans and tests that are part of clinical trial protocols, should be discussed with patients and family caregivers as part of treatment decision making.

DISCUSSING BENEFITS AND BURDENS OF CONTINUING CANCER TREATMENT NEAR THE END OF LIFE

Studies from the United States and other developed nations over the past 30 years continue to confirm that cancer patients, when faced with decisions about chemotherapy offering a small chance of prolonging life by a few weeks to a few months, and with the certainty of toxic side effects, will tend to continue treatment (Matsuyama, Reddy, & Smith, 2006). At some point, the hopes invested in "treatment" may crowd out adequate consideration of what can be hoped *for* from any potential treatment.

The responsible professional should help patients and families to think clearly about each decision concerning whether to start, continue, or stop treatment. Professionals who treat patients living with advanced cancer may themselves grapple with uncertainty over the value of continuing chemotherapy due to factors such as an individual patient's history of responsiveness to therapy, their own clinical observations concerning the effectiveness of newer therapies, and encouraging reports from ongoing clinical trials. While it may be easier to continue to order another round of treatment or switch to another regimen rather than to frankly discuss prognosis, professionals should address prognosis and options when further treatment may offer more burdens than benefits. There must be a potential physiological benefit to any cancer treatment regimen proposed to a patient or family: Treatment should not be used simply to be "doing something." If the patient or family inquires about a treatment that has no potential for benefit, the responsible professional should explain why this treatment is not an option for this patient. This is much easier to do if a relationship of trust has been developed over the course of an advance-care-planning and goal-setting process.

Oncologists and other health care professionals who see patients with advanced cancer in the community setting, including private practice as well as a hospital's outpatient clinics, may be unsure about raising the option of forgoing further efforts to intervene in the course of the disease and shifting the focus to relieving pain and symptoms through palliative care or hospice enrollment. Because these professionals typically see patients in the context of treatment appointments, it may feel awkward to broach the topic of hospice.

Having an advance-care-planning process in place within a practice or clinic will facilitate these conversations by ensuring that patients have already had an opportunity to discuss and document their goals of care, and that patients whose diagnoses indicate that they are hospice-eligible receive accurate information about the Medicare hospice benefit. In the absence of a formal institutional process, oncologists who see patients outside of the hospital setting should be prepared to initiate treatment decision-making discussions, including the option to forgo treatment and transition to hospice care, with patients and families.

Cancer patients who are receiving treatment outside of a hospital setting may have difficulty gaining access to palliative care services that are organized around inpatient consultations. Oncologists, nurse practitioners, and nurses who treat cancer patients in the community have a special responsibility to determine how their patients' needs for pain and symptom management and supportive care can be met. Clinicians who are affiliated with a cancer center should find out how their center's palliative care service can meet the needs of outpatients. Clinicians in private practice may need to seek out additional training in pain and symptom management and to add a palliative care orientation to the treatment of their patients, including those with advanced disease.

PROFESSIONALS WITHOUT BORDERS: AN ETHIC OF COLLABORATION FOR CANCER CARE PROVIDERS

Ethical dilemmas are often described as occurring in a "gray area," where moral actions are not clearly right or wrong. The care of patients with advanced cancer contains many gray areas, many places where sharp distinctions— between treatment and research, between therapeutic treatment and palliative treatment, between hospital and hospice, between the process of living with a chronic illness and the process of dying from a progressive illness—have become blurred. These gray areas can be confusing and stressful places for patients, families, and professionals alike, in part because the story of what chronicity means in cancer, and with respect to different types of cancer, is not yet clear. Also unclear are the ethical obligations that come with being a professional who cares for persons with chronic cancer. The culture of oncology is still a culture that aims to cure disease, and that is a laudable goal. When disease cannot be cured, when the goal is control, the relationship between oncologist and patient must encompass the discussion of both clinical information and treatment options and other, less tangible, topics: hopes; fears; coping with the impact of cancer on a patient's body, relationships, income, and identity; learning how to adapt to continual changes resulting from a disease that resists stability.

The border between chronic disease and progressive, eventually terminal, disease may be discernible only in retrospect. A patient with advanced disease whose treatment is aimed at managing pain and symptoms may have a better quality of life than a patient with advanced disease who is still benefiting from therapy aimed at preventing progression but is experiencing significant treatment-induced burdens. Both of these patients are living with cancer; both may be hospice-eligible; both should have access to optimal palliative care whether or not they choose to enroll in hospice. When a region's natural borders cannot be discerned, efforts to impose them artificially may work against the interests of the people who have to live there. The politics of the region called advanced cancer are complex. Professionals who have chosen to work there should recognize a mutual ethical obligation to collaborate with one another, across institutions and healthcare settings, in the interests of those who will live in this region for the rest of their lives.

Nancy Berlinger, PhD, MDiv, is deputy director and research scholar at the Hastings Center, a bioethics research institute in Garrison, New York. Her research interests include end-of-life care; palliative care; ethics and policy in chronic cancer; ethics in healthcare chaplaincy; and patient safety and quality improvement. Dr. Berlinger is the author of After Harm: Medical Error and the Ethics of Forgiveness, *and project director of the forthcoming revision of the Hastings Center guidelines on end-of-life care. She is an instructor in healthcare ethics at Yale School of Nursing.*

Bruce Jennings is director of the Center for Humans and Nature, a private foundation that supports work on environmental and public health policy and planning. He is also senior consultant to the Hastings Center and teaches at the Yale School of Public Health. He has written or edited 20 books and has published more than 150 articles on bioethics and public policy issues. He is currently working on new ethical guidelines on end-of-life care under development at the Hastings Center.

REFERENCES

Abelson, R. (2007, February 10). A chance to pick hospice, and still hope to live. *New York Times*, Business section, National edition.

Appelbaum, P. S., Roth, L. H., Lidz, C. W., Benson, P., & Winslade, W. (1987). False hopes and best data: Consent to research and the therapeutic misconception. *Hastings Center Report, 17*(2), 20–24.

Bodenheimer, T., Lorig, K., Holman, H., & Grumbach, K. (2002). Patient self-management of chronic disease in primary care. *Journal of the American Medical Association, 288*(19), 2469–2475.

Dufresne, A., Pivot, X., Tournigand, C., Facchini, T., Altweegg, T., Chaigneau, L., et al. (2008). Impact of chemotherapy beyond the first line in patients with metastatic breast cancer. *Breast Cancer Research and Treatment, 107*(2), 275–279.

Fojo, T., & Grady, C. (2009). How much is life worth: Cetuximab, non-small cell lung cancer, and the $440 billion question. *Journal of the National Cancer Institute, 101*(15), 1–5.

Glynne-Jones, R., Ostler, P., Lumley-Graybow, S., Chait, I., Hughes, R., Grainger, J., et al. (2006). Can I look at my list? An evaluation of a 'prompt sheet' within an oncology outpatient clinic. *Clinical Oncology, 18*(5), 395–400.

Harrington, S. E., & Smith, T. J. (2008). The role of chemotherapy at the end of life: When is enough, enough? *Journal of the American Medical Association, 299*(22), 2667–2678.

Hillner, B. E., & Smith, T. J. (2009). Efficacy does not necessarily translate to cost effectiveness: A case study in the challenges associated with 21st-century cancer drug pricing. *Journal of Clinical Oncology, 27*(13), 2111–2113.

Jennings, B., Caplan, A., & Callahan, D. (1988). Ethical challenges of chronic illness. *Hastings Center Report, 18*(1), 1–16.

Matsuyama, R., Reddy, S., & Smith, T. J. (2006). Why do patients choose chemotherapy near the end of life? A review of the perspective of those facing death from cancer. *Journal of Clinical Oncology, 24*(21), 3490–3496.

National Comprehensive Cancer Network. (2008). Task force report on oral chemotherapy. *Journal of the National Comprehensive Cancer Network, 6*(Suppl. 3), S1–S14.

National Hospice and Palliative Care Organization. (2008). *Hospice facts and figures: Hospice care in America* (p. 8). Arlington, VA: Author. Available at http://www.nhpco.org/files/public/Statistics_Research/NHPCO_facts-and-figures_2008.pdf

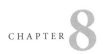

The Transition to Palliative Care

Brad Stuart

Throughout the Western world, the last half of the 20th century witnessed unprecedented progress in biological science and innovation in health care technology. Although mortality rates had been decreasing since the 1800s, after the development of antibiotics during World War II, mortality rates began to drop more rapidly. By the close of the century, for the first time in their 50,000-year history, humans had taken their lives, and their life expectancies, into their own hands.

The advent of the 21st century, however, has brought new challenges. As the Baby Boom generation edges into Medicare eligibility, as chronic illness assumes a dominant role as the primary cause of mortality, and as health care costs reach levels that threaten economic development, questions have arisen about the indiscriminate use of medical technology. In particular, intensive and expensive treatment near the end of life has become controversial.

TREATMENT AT THE END OF LIFE: WHAT BENEFIT?

By many measures, health care in the United States provided to patients near death is increasingly aggressive. More than one quarter of all Medicare dollars are spent in the last year of patients' lives. Of this, 40% is spent in the last month before death, of which 80% goes for hospital treatment (Centers for Medicare and Medicaid Services, 2003). Clearly, our health care system places a high premium on fighting death—and, some might say, on denying it.

Although most people, including most physicians, assume that aggressive treatment prolongs life, research shows that this is not necessarily true. There is marked variation in treatment intensity and cost in the last 2 years of life across the United States. In the most expensive regions, up to 60% more intensive care unit (ICU) days, specialty inpatient consults, tests, and procedures are provided compared with the most economical areas. However, this extra spending produces no better mortality rates, access to care, quality of life, or patient satisfaction (Fisher et al., 2003). In other words, more aggressive treatment is not better.

Cancer treatment in particular is becoming more aggressive over time. For example, in non-small-cell lung cancer (NSCLC), intensive care near the end of life, often with mechanical ventilation, is now common practice. In a study by Reichner, Thompson, O'Brien, Kuru, and Anderson (2006), 74% of NSCLC patients sent to the ICU were "full-code" on admission. However, intensive care provided little benefit. Seventy-four percent of ventilated NSCLC patients, an identical proportion, died before they could leave the unit.

Sharma, Freeman, Zhang, and Goodwin (2008) reported that in a study of 45,627 Medicare fee-for-service patients with advanced lung cancer in the Surveillance, Epidemiology, and End-Results (SEER) database from 1993 to 2002, hospital costs for ICU-admitted patients were 114% higher ($25,929 vs. $12,133) than those for patients treated on the ward. The ICU admission accounted for 80% of terminal hospitalization costs. Yet the average gain in life expectancy from ICU admission—33 days—was no better than that seen with hospice care. However, hospice enrollees with lung cancer survive, on average, 39 days longer than patients who undergo cancer treatment (Connor, Pyenson, Fitch, Spence, & Iwasake, 2007). The same is true for almost all other diagnostic groups in hospice. Ironically, although it is counterintuitive to most patients, families, and physicians, the best way to keep the most seriously ill patients alive may be not to send them to the ICU, but to send them to hospice.

THE TRANSITION TO PALLIATIVE CARE

As options for aggressive care have multiplied, the transition from disease-modifying treatment to palliative care has become more challenging. Easy access to hospital care whenever patients are ill, especially because health insurance shields them from awareness of its high costs, has led to expectations that hospital care should and will be provided whenever patients' conditions worsen. Agreeing to withdrawal of treatment is not easy for many patients and families because it feels like giving up, it implies impending death to patients, and it triggers fear of abandonment by the medical profession (Baile, Glober, Lenzi, Beale, & Kudelka, 1999). Unfortunately, these fears may be well founded. Many physicians also have trouble stopping treatment and supporting transition to palliative care, and when they do stop treatment, some may terminate their relationship with the patient and family.

Medical technology's success in raising life expectancy has also raised society's expectations. Some people's beliefs are challenged by research showing that more treatment is not better and that advance care planning and referral to palliative care is beneficial. Political debate surrounding health care reform bears this out. Pro-reform advocates quote study results, but opponents counter with accusations that reform will reduce access to care and lead to the death of large numbers of seniors. Policy change that reduces inappropriate use of high-tech medicine for patients near the end of life, or that incentivizes end-of-life care, may not emerge from this debate. Even as reimbursement is reduced, physicians, patients, and families will most likely have to decide what kind of care is best—as they do now.

THE PRIMACY OF EMOTION

Parker et al. (2001) reported that technical expertise ranks first among qualities patients want in their oncologists. However, when it comes to changing goals toward palliative care, other factors are important. No matter how clear the research findings are, data alone do not change minds. Issues of life and death affect people on a deep emotional level, beneath rationality. Ultimately, on both the policy and the personal levels, health care decisions are made on the basis of emotional considerations. Reason plays a role, but feelings, which are often unconscious, often trump the intellect.

Even though many patients state that their quality of life should be the dominant value in decision making as illness advances, this conviction often gets disregarded. Jansen et al. (2001) found that almost 40% of breast cancer patients on chemotherapy would continue it, even if there was no clinical benefit at all and no additional chance for survival. Likewise, in cases where the benefits of chemotherapy were doubtful (and therefore the physician would have to tell the patient that the disease was likely fatal), oncologists offered it anyway, stating that "doing something," i.e., giving chemotherapy, was preferable to "doing nothing" by providing supportive care (de Haes & Koedoot, 2003). Medical training and economic factors, which can color doctors' feelings and attitudes about their practice, are also influential. One physician said, "Giving chemotherapy, rather than watchful waiting, is what I have been educated to do; it's what I have to sell in my shop."

Neuroscience tells us that emotion actually plays a major, but not necessarily conscious, role in reason and decision making. Descartes may have celebrated the intellect (and split the mind from the body) when he declared, "I think, therefore I am," but in reality the brain uses emotion to think things through and to decide what is best for the body.

Emotions are a two-edged sword: They help the decision-making process when participants are conscious enough to make use of them, but they can interfere if they remain unconscious. Doctors may make better, more patient-centered decisions when they become aware of their feelings so that their thinking is not run by them. Neuroscientist Antonio Damasio (1994) observes,

> All great physicians have been those men and women who are not only well versed in the hard-core physiopathology of their time, but are equally at ease, mostly through their own insight and accumulated wisdom, with the human heart in conflict. Yet we would be deluding ourselves if we thought that the standard of medical practice in the Western world is that of the notable physicians we all have known.

Indeed, the physicians who appear to be able to help most with the transition to palliative care are those who are familiar and comfortable with issues related to "the human heart in conflict." Jackson et al. (2008), in a study of 18 academic oncologists and the emotions they experience, found that only 25% of these doctors reported that their conception of care included both biomedical and psychosocial aspects. They had a clearer communication strategy, an ability to positively influence patient and family coping with and accepting the dying process, and success in aiding the transition from treatment to palliation. In contrast, cancer specialists who viewed their role as primarily biomedical reported more-distant patient relationships, a sense of failure at their inability to alter the course of disease, inability to affect patient/family coping or acceptance, and unwillingness to make recommendations about end-of-life treatment options.

Many oncologists, even those who see themselves as emotionally aware, avoid feelings in discussions with patients. Pollack et al. (2007) recorded almost 400 clinic discussions among 51 oncologists and 270 patients with advanced cancer; they found that physicians created openings for emotional expression by patients in only 37% of conversations. This small number of "empathic opportunities" elicited a feeling response from physicians only 22% of the time; in the remainder the doctor changed the subject with a "terminator statement" related to the medical details of the case. This behavior was largely unconscious: Most of the oncologists expressed high confidence in their ability to address patients' concerns and believed that addressing emotions would benefit patients. Sixty-one percent of the oncologists had received some kind of communication training.

CHALLENGES IN COMMUNICATION

Conversations between physicians and patients about upcoming end-of-life issues are critical to the success of transitions to palliative care. Zhang et al. (2009) reported that patients with advanced cancer who stated that they had talked to their physicians about the possibility of dying had fewer aggressive interventions and incurred lower costs of care. Conversely, patients who did not have such conversations had more days in intensive care and more invasive procedures like intubation and mechanical ventilation, and the quality of their dying was worse.

The transition to palliative care should take place in a context of shared decision making between patient/family and clinicians, usually physicians. To make plans, patients and their surrogates need information about the disease process; what to expect over the course of their illness; their likely prognosis; and their options for care, particularly hospice.

Imparting this information, especially when it contains "bad news" about prognosis that patients might find alarming, has proven challenging for physicians for several reasons. First, prognosis is difficult for doctors. They feel poorly prepared to do it, they feel patients and colleagues expect an unreasonable degree of certainty, they feel they might be judged if they are wrong, and they do not agree on what constitutes a terminal state (Christakis & Iwashyna, 1998). These factors combine to produce a general reluctance among doctors to formulate prognoses and state them to patients and families. Physicians report that even if they were asked by patients, they would conceal the truth or consciously over- or understate prognostic estimates, in almost two thirds of cases (Lamont & Christakis, 2001). When they do provide prognostic estimates, physicians tend to overestimate the time patients have left to live by a factor of 5.3 (Christakis & Lamont, 2000). These barriers to the transition from treatment to palliation cause, in the opinions of doctors themselves, inappropriately late referrals to hospice and palliative care (Christakis & Iwashyna, 2000).

COMMUNICATION PROTOCOLS

Guidelines have been published and widely disseminated for communication about terminal prognosis from clinicians to patients and families. These protocols have become a mainstay in palliative care education, despite the fact that there has been little research to support their effectiveness because of methodological difficulties in studying them (Eggly et al., 2006).

The most commonly used communication system is included in the Education for Physicians on End-of-Life Care (EPEC) curriculum (Emanuel, Von Gunten, & Ferris, 1999). Module Two contains a six-step protocol for delivering bad news. The EPEC protocol is in turn adapted from the SPIKES model (Baile et al., 2000), consisting of six steps:

- *Setting*: creating the best physical circumstances for the meeting; deciding on participants; ensuring accurate understanding of clinical facts of the case
- *Perception*: ascertaining the patient's understanding of the situation using "ask before you tell" methods
- *Invitation*: ascertaining how much and what kind of information the patient wants to hear regarding disease and prognosis
- *Knowledge*: imparting clinical impressions and supporting data that constitute "bad news"; using nontechnical language; coming into alignment with the patient
- *Empathy*: eliciting honest emotional reactions from the patient and other participants; responding with empathy and active listening; ensuring that the patient feels heard
- *Strategy/Summary*: assembling plans for next steps in care

DISCUSSING THE TRANSITION

A review of evidence-based findings about how to facilitate the transition from curative to palliative care has been published by Schofield, Carey, Love, Nehill, and Wein (2006). Most of the evidence is descriptive, as only three systematic reviews of randomized trials were identified. Pain is the most common trigger for referral to palliative care. During the discussion, most people want information on the disease process and their prognosis; the small number of exceptions include older patients and those whose disease is very advanced. Most patients tend to underestimate the extent of their disease and, like their physicians, to be overly optimistic about their prognosis. Communication about fatal disease must be explicit, with checking to make sure patients heard the facts. Fried, Bradley, and O'Leary (2003) found that only 20% of patients said that the doctor told them that their disease was fatal; in 49% of the cases, the clinicians felt they had said this, but the patients stated they hadn't heard. Misperceptions are important, because patients who are inappropriately optimistic tend to ask for futile treatment (Weeks et al., 1998).

Up to 90% of patients want to know their chances of cure and all possible treatment options. Evasion or dishonesty may cause or add to patients' distress (Fallowfield, Jenkins, & Beveridge, 2002), as does doctors' unwillingness to explore family members' feelings (Morita et al., 2004). Helpful interventions include the following:

- *Eliciting patients' concerns*: Ask what patients are concerned about emotionally, especially their fears, whether or not a therapeutic solution exists. Physicians have traditionally been taught that the way to help patients is to fix their problems; they may believe that asking about feelings that can't be fixed is inappropriate or useless. In reality, research shows that simply expressing concerns can deactivate them, improving symptom control (Smyth, Stone, Hurewitz, & Kaell, 1999). Unless the clinician asks, most patients will not bring up their concerns, particularly if they are anxious or depressed (Heaven & Maguire, 1997).
- *Empathy*: Acknowledge feelings when they are expressed. Empathy can be conveyed by naming the emotion, making sure the patient realizes that it is understood, showing respect for the patient's ability to cope, letting the patient know support will be there no matter what happens, and asking open-ended questions to explore other aspects of experience (Smith & Hoppe, 1991).
- *Active listening*: Simply summarize what has been said, altering the patient's wording slightly, to make sure patients and family members know their feelings were heard. This is especially important in response to requests for futile treatment, when inadequately understood, expressed, or acknowledged feelings of terror or desperation may be a motivating force.
- *"Ask-tell-ask"*: Find out what the patient knows and feels before giving information, then check for comprehension. This allows the clinician first to get on the patient's "wavelength," to understand how best to express difficult concepts in terms the patient can understand. Then the information can be given and patient/family perceptions can be checked to make sure important points were heard and understood.
- *"I wish" statements*: Respond to denial of difficult news or requests for futile treatment by stating, "I wish it could be different." This emphasizes the reality of the situation, even when patients want to deny or disregard it, and puts the patient, family, and clinician on the same side of the table (Ptacek & Eberhardt, 1996).

- *Hope for the best, prepare for the worst*: Establish realistic goals that allow for hope, even if it seems unrealistic, but still make good plans. Hoping for a cure, even if it is unlikely, is not the real problem. Worse is ignoring real possibilities for action. It is reasonable to hope for cure, but prudent to do advance care planning and take care of financial issues in case problems do arise.

BALANCING REALISM AND HOPE

Underlying the reluctance both patients and clinicians feel about discussing end-of-life issues is the possibility that hope may be lost. Hearing that disease is incurable and that death is likely, even if it is far off in the future, has an emotional impact that can be devastating. Hopelessness is a state that most people dread and therefore avoid if at all possible. Redefining hope, and helping it to evolve as death approaches, is a key to helping with the transition (Evans, Tulsky, Back, & Arnold, 2006).

It is important to make a distinction between appropriate hope and false hope. Fostering false hope, or colluding in it with patients and families who are grasping for any hint of good news, may result in failed expectations and regret over lost opportunities to live fully with whatever time people have together. Appropriate hope focuses on what can actually be done in real life, whether the disease can be cured or not. Clayton, Butow, Arnold, and Tattersall (2005) found that patients feel it is possible for clinicians to foster coping skills and nurture hope while discussing even poor prognoses and end-of-life issues. Even bad news helps people cope better than no news because it reduces uncertainty, which promotes worries about imagined outcomes that can be worse than the ones that are likely to happen.

Humans are extremely adaptable and, with support, can adjust to situations that might seem intolerable to others. The key for clinicians is to leave space, in their own awareness and in their relationship with patients, for hope to evolve, as it often does near the end of life. Remarkable transformations can happen when patients learn to face what they had been afraid to contemplate, and as they begin to trust enough to let go of the control that may have seemed indispensable before. As the end of life nears for many patients and families, hope becomes irrelevant because life in the present moment is all that is needed.

CONCLUSION

The transition from curative treatment for cancer to palliative care has become more important as options for care have increased, along with costs. Barriers to this transition often center on emotional issues, many of which are not fully conscious, on the part of patients, families, and physicians. Better communication that attends to the emotional content of discussions about disease process, prognosis, and options for care would help with advance care planning and the transition to palliative care.

REFERENCES

Baile, W., Buckman, R., Lenzi, R., Blober, G., Beale E., & Kudelka, A. (2000). SPIKES – A six-step protocol for delivering bad news: Application to the patient with cancer. *Oncologist, 5*, 302–311.

Baile, W. F., Glober, G. A., Lenzi, R., Beale, E. A., & Kudelka, A. P. (1999). Discussing disease progression and end-of-life decisions. *Oncology, 13*, 1021–1027.

Centers for Medicare and Medicaid Services, Office of Research, Development, and Information. (2003, May). Last year of life expenditures. *MCBS Profiles*, no. 10.

Christakis, N. A., & Iwashyna, T. J. (1998). Attitude and self-reported practice regarding prognostication in a national sample of internists. *Archives of Internal Medicine, 158*, 2389–2395.

Christakis, N. A., & Iwashyna, T. J. (2000). The impact of individual and market factors on the timing of initiation of hospice terminal care. *Medical Care, 38*, 528–541.

Christakis, N. A., & Lamont, E. B. (2000). Extent and determinants of error in doctors' prognoses in terminally-ill patients: Prospective cohort study. *BMJ, 320*, 469–473.

Clayton, J. M., Butow, P. N., Arnold, R. M., & Tattersall, M. H. N. (2005). Fostering coping and nurturing hope when discussing the future with terminally ill cancer patients and their caregivers. *Cancer, 103*, 1965–1975.

Connor, S. R., Pyenson, B., Fitch, K., Spence, C., & Iwasake, K. (2007). Comparing hospice and non-hospice patient survival among patients who die within a three-year window. *Journal of Pain and Symptom Management, 33*, 238–246.

Damasio, A. R. (1994). *Descartes' error: Emotion, reason, and the human brain* (p. 257). New York: Avon Books.

De Haes, H., & Koedoot, N. (2003). Patient-centered decision making in palliative care treatment: A world of paradoxes. *Patient Education and Counseling, 50,* 43–49.

Eggly, S., Penner, L., Albrecht, T., Cline, R., Foster, T., et al. (2006). Discussing bad news in the outpatient oncology clinic: Rethinking current communication guidelines. *Journal of Clinical Oncology, 24,* 716–719.

Emanuel, L. L., Von Gunten, C. F., & Ferris, F. D. (Eds.). (1999). *The EPEC curriculum: Education for physicians on end-of-life care.* Retrieved July 27, 2009, from http://www.epec.net/EPEC/Webpages/index.cfm

Evans, W. G., Tulsky, J. A., Back, A. L., & Arnold, R. M. (2006). Communication at times of transitions: How to help patients cope with loss and redefine hope. *Cancer Journal, 12,* 417–424.

Fallowfield, L. J., Jenkins, V. A., & Beveridge, H. A. (2002). Truth may hurt but deceit hurts more: Communication in palliative care. *Palliative Medicine, 16,* 297–303.

Fisher, E. S., Wennberg, D. E., Stukel, T. A., Gottlieb, D. J., Lucas, F. L., & Pinder, E. L. (2003). The implications of regional variations in Medicare spending. Part 2: Health outcomes and satisfaction with care. *Annals of Internal Medicine, 138,* 288–298.

Fried, T. R., Bradley, E. H., & O'Leary, J. (2003). Prognosis communication in serious illness: Perceptions of older patients, caregivers, and clinicians. *Journal of the American Geriatrics Society, 51,* 1398–1403.

Heaven, C. M., & Maguire, P. (1997). Disclosure of concerns by hospice patients and their identification by nurses. *Palliative Medicine, 11,* 283–290.

Jackson, V. A., Mack, J., Matsuyama, R., Lakoma, M. D., Sullivan, A. M., et al. (2008). A qualitative study of oncologists' approaches to end-of-life care. *Journal of Palliative Medicine, 11,* 893–903.

Jansen, S. J. T., Kievit, J., Nooij, M. A., de Haes, J. C. J. M., Overpelt, I. M. E., et al. (2001). Patients' preferences for adjuvant chemotherapy in early-stage breast cancer: Is treatment worthwhile? *British Journal of Cancer, 84,* 1577–1585.

Lamont, E. B., & Christakis, N. A. (2001). Prognostic disclosure to patients with cancer near the end of life. *Annals of Internal Medicine, 134,* 1096–1105.

Morita, T., Akechi, T., Ikenaga, M., Kizawa Y., Kohara, H., et al. (2004). Communication about the ending of anticancer treatment and transition to palliative care. *Annals of Oncology, 15,* 1551–1557.

Parker, P. A., Baile, W. F., DeMoor, C., Lenzi, R., Kudelka, A. P., & Cohen, L. (2001). Breaking bad news about cancer: Patients' preferences for communication. *Journal of Clinical Oncology, 19,* 2049–2056.

Pollack, K. I., Arnold, R. M., Jeffrys, A. S., Alexander, S. C., Olsen, M. K., et al. (2007). Oncologist communication about emotion during visits with patients with advanced cancer. *Journal of Clinical Oncology, 25,* 5748–5752.

Ptacek, J. T., & Eberhardt, T. L. (1996). Breaking bad news: A review of the literature. *JAMA, 276,* 496–502.

Reichner, C. A., Thompson, J. A., O'Brien, S., Kuru, T., & Anderson, E. D. (2006). Outcome and code status of lung cancer patients admitted to the medical ICU. *Chest, 130,* 719–723.

Schofield, P., Carey, M., Love, A., Nehill, C., & Wein, S. (2006). "Would you like to talk about your future treatment options?" Discussing the transition from curative cancer treatment to palliative care. *Palliative Medicine, 20,* 397–406.

Sharma, G., Freeman, J., Zhang, D., & Goodwin, J. S. (2008). Trends in end-of-life ICU use among older adults with advanced lung cancer. *Chest, 133,* 72–78.

Smith, R. C., & Hoppe, R. B. (1991). The patient's story: Integrating patient- and physician-centered approaches in interviewing. *Annals of Internal Medicine, 115,* 470–477.

Smyth, J. M., Stone, A. A., Hurewitz, A., & Kaell, A. (1999). Effects of writing about stressful experiences on symptom reduction in patients with asthma or rheumatoid arthritis: A randomized trial. *JAMA, 281,* 1304–1309.

Weeks, J. C., Cook, E. F., O'Day, S. J., Peterson, L. M., Wenger, N., et al. (1998). Relationship between cancer patients' predictions of prognosis and their treatment preferences. *JAMA, 279,* 1709–1714.

Zhang, B., Wright, A. A., Huskamp, H. A., Nilsson, M. E., Maciejewski, M. L., et al. (2009). Health care costs in the last week of life: Associations with end-of-life conversations. *Archives of Internal Medicine, 169,* 480–488.

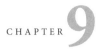

End-Stage Cancer: The Role of Palliative Care and Hospice

Sherry R. Schachter

A t some point as cancer patients continue along the dying trajectory, they realize that they are no longer winning their fight against cancer. Although cure no longer seems probable, they frequently remain hopeful for what they want for themselves (Winterling, Wasteson, Glimelius, Sjoden, & Nordin, 2004; Doka, 1993). They may hope to be surrounded by loved ones and not die alone or they may hope to die in a hospital where they are just a call bell away from the medical staff and pain relief. They may hope to see a grandchild's first communion or the birth of a great-grandchild. They may hope to die in their sleep, unaware of what may be happening. Whatever the course of their journey has been, the experience of living with a life-threatening illness has been unique to them and their family. Although similarities may exist, each one travels the road in his or her own way, determined by personality, life experience, core beliefs, past coping techniques, and ultimately, inner strength to face the difficult decisions that determine one's course of action at the end of life.

Making the decision to forgo active curative therapy in favor of aggressive palliative therapy is not done easily or without struggle. It is common for those who have aggressively sought second, third, and even fourth opinions and those who have struggled with alternative therapies along with conventional courses of treatment to feel that they have failed in their battle against cancer. Despite the knowledge we have gained since Dr. Cicely Saunders opened St. Christopher's Hospice in Great Britain in 1967, there is national and even worldwide confusion as to the philosophical underpinnings of hospice and palliative care (Connor, 2009). This deficiency in our knowledge is pertinent to healthcare professionals, patients, and families—evidenced by the untimeliness of physician referrals to hospice. Unfortunately, research indicates that the median length of stay in a hospice program is less than 20 days (Connor, 2009).

Any life-threatening illness is a family illness as it affects the entire family (Schachter, 2009). Patients and families have similar needs as they face daunting physical, spiritual, social, and psychological challenges at the end of life (Corr, 1991; Doka, 1993). Dr. Michael Brescia, medical director of Calvary Hospital (New York), has repeatedly described the process of metastases by asking audiences, "Where is the first place lung cancer metastases to?" The answer: the family. If a patient has lung cancer, the entire family has lung cancer.

Although unique differences exist in the way people cope with end-of-life issues, there are also similarities in that all patients face medical, ethical, existential, and psychological issues that may determine the course of their decisions and ultimately impact their death.

MEDICAL ISSUES AND CONCERNS

There are several obstacles hindering a patient's decision to terminate aggressive medical treatment and consider palliative care and hospice. One is the need to preserve hope (Schachter, 2009). Inaugurating the discussion of end-of-life palliative care must center on the recognition that there is no "one right way" and no "one right place" to die (Schachter & Coyle, 1998), wherever that care is delivered (e.g., home, hospital, hospice, or nursing home). Clear, concise, and open communication is a potent tool in initiating and maintaining effective interventions for end-of-life care. The dialogue between patients, family caregivers, and physicians is challenging when trying to preserve hope. As the disease progresses and the patient's condition deteriorates, patients and physicians often avoid discussions about end-of-life care or the presence of discouraging statistics. Instead, their conversations may focus on the curative potential of a procedure (Lee, Fairclough, Antin, & Woods, 2001). Miyaji (1993) and Weeks et al. (1998) noted that physicians tend to withhold or minimize some pertinent information and often change the language they used when communicating with their patients because they fear that patients will become distressed and lose hope. Miyaji found that two thirds of physicians modify the information given to patients when they think that the truth "will have a seriously bad outcome." Seeking to preserve a patient's sense of hope was a central reason for doctors to soften the impact of giving bad news, even if it meant withholding information to help the patient maintain a positive attitude (Friedrichsen & Strang, 2003).

Yet, after death, bereaved family members frequently report that they never realized death was imminent and that their loved one was dying. For these bereaved family members, maintaining hope was viewed as critical for both them and their dying loved one. A discussion about hospice or palliative care would have been viewed as "giving up" and admitting defeat.

While honest, open communication between the physician and the dying patient is necessary, so too is the physician's ability to accurately assess the patient's prognosis and life span and then continue to have that discussion in a timely manner. This is crucial for many reasons, including the criteria for hospice admission that patients have a prognosis of 6 months or less and be willing to forgo therapy aimed at a cure (United States Department of Health and Human Services, 2000). Late patient admission into a hospice program can create financial, clinical, and emotional problems for both healthcare providers and the patient (Christakis, 1994). A study by Mackillop and Quirt (1997) asked oncologists to (1) predict the likelihood of a cure for cancer patients receiving ambulatory treatment; and (2) estimate the survival rates for those cancer patients they identified as having no possible likelihood of cure. Results showed that although the physicians in the study were accurate at predicting which patients would most likely be cured, they were not successful in predicting survival rates, and were able to do so for only one third of the patients.

Physicians may find giving their patients bad news difficult because of their own denial and discomfort. It has been suggested that the physician's own anxiety affects the way his or her patient is informed of the cancer diagnosis and overall prognosis (Righetti & Giorgio, 1994).

The major SUPPORT study produced several sobering findings including the following: (1) more than half of physicians were unaware of what kind of care their patients preferred for life-sustaining treatment; (2) severe pain was common in dying patients, with half having moderate to severe pain at least half of the time before their death; and (3) nearly 40% of patients spent at least 10 days in intensive care units hooked up to machines before they died (SUPPORT Principal Investigators, 1995). Recent studies in hospice and palliative care indicate that death does not have to be characterized by uncontrollable pain and that hospice teams are successful at accurately assessing, managing, and relieving the pain and suffering of dying patients (Connor, 2009).

The following case scenario illustrates examples of things gone wrong, as well as a positive experience once the decision was made for hospice care.

CASE STUDY

Emily had been a vibrant 58-year-old woman diagnosed with inoperable non-small-cell lung cancer the year before. She had undergone several rounds of radiation and chemotherapy. Initially, her husband did not like or trust physicians, social workers, and health providers in general. He tried to manage his wife's medications himself and often discontinued medications without notifying the nurses. "The medical profession only wants to knock her out. All they worry about is her pain. They don't care about her communicating with me" (Schachter, 1999). Emily's pain became severe and persistent accompanied by intractable hiccups that affected her quality of life. Several months before her death, Emily was admitted into a hospice program where her pain was finally controlled and well managed. Her husband had remained adamant about not having his wife sedated and wanted her to be alert and awake at home. The hospice team was successfully able to manage that very fine balance between managing the patient's pain yet having her awake and a participant in her care. This was a turning point for the patient's husband who began to trust the hospice team members. He no longer tried to manage Emily's medications and although he continued to refuse spiritual care, he was accepting of the emotional support that was offered. When Emily died, she died peacefully at home with her husband at her side.

How and when one makes the transition from aggressive curative treatment to aggressive palliative and hospice care is dependent on many factors. For some people, the fear of pain, suffering, and distressing symptoms may push them to quickly accept care aimed at ameliorating these distressing symptoms. For others, an awareness of the changes occurring within the body may make the realization of their prognosis more immediate and alarming. For others, the decision to enroll in a hospice program may come with the realization that they can no longer take care of themselves.

ETHICAL ISSUES AND CONCERNS

Legal and ethical issues at the end of life are multifaceted and complex. For many people in the United States, having and maintaining control is the primary focus of their being. Yet decisions about end-of-life care can and should be initiated prior to an emergency situation. Open, frank discussions between the patient, family members or significant others, and the physician assure that the patient's wishes will be heard, understood, and respected. Goals of care need to be fully discussed and appropriate documentation completed to ensure compliance.

Advance directives are instructions given by individuals specifying what actions should be taken in the event that they are no longer able to make decisions due to illness or incapacity.

Before completing these documents, the patient should give thought to his or her preferences regarding artificial nutrition and hydration, kidney dialysis, use of antibiotics or blood transfusions, organ donation, etc. Because these decisions should be made before a medical crisis occurs, thought should also be given to different kinds of death—not just a cancer death. Are these the decisions I would want if I had Alzheimer's disease or if I were in a permanent coma? What are my beliefs and wishes about resuscitation? Do-not-resuscitate orders? It is important for patients to keep their family members apprised of their wishes—whether or not a certain family member is the designated proxy—because it clarifies the patient's beliefs and helps prevent family conflicts. Hospice chaplain Hank Dunn has written about the difficulties and struggles siblings frequently encounter when making end-of-life decisions for their elderly parents. Even if they share ethical, medical, or religious opinions on withholding or withdrawing treatment, they may be worlds apart emotionally (Dunn, n.d.). These charged emotions at the end of life can impact coping skills and ultimately bereavement outcomes after the death.

CASE STUDY

Bob was a youthful 72-year-old widowed professor who 10 years prior had survived a myocardial infarction. After his long recuperation, he prepared his living will and designated his youngest daughter as his healthcare proxy. Bob put much thought into these two documents as he considered who would be making medical decisions for him and what future medical care he wanted and did not want. His prior close call with mortality paved the way for him to become proactive in preparing for his future. However, Bob had been estranged from another daughter and did not share his thoughts or wishes with her or inform her of his decisions. Later, while being actively treated for prostate cancer he suffered a cerebrovascular accident (stroke) and became paralyzed and unable to articulate his wishes. Knowing her father's wishes, the daughter refused any intravenous administration and the placement of a feeding tube. Although the healthcare proxy ultimately could and did make decisions that were legally binding, numerous arguments between the two siblings created hard feelings and impacted the grieving process for both daughters after Bob's death.

Another aid in end-of-life planning is the preparation of an ethical will. Writing an ethical will encourages the dying patient to share his or her wisdom with loved ones; thoughts and reflections of the past; and dreams the dying person has for their future. This personal legacy can be a gift for those who are bereaved.

CASE STUDY

Jackie was a 49-year-old woman diagnosed with colon cancer. She had three children, ranging in age from 11 to 21 years. Jackie began to write a journal and letters for her children, believing it would be her legacy to her family. She started writing her journal at the time of her diagnosis and continued until a week before her death. Everything she wrote, she wrote consciously and purposefully, knowing that after her death the journals would be read and interpreted by her loved ones. She wrote of her dreams for them and what she would want for them to achieve in their life.

SPIRITUAL/EXISTENTIAL ISSUES AND CONCERNS

Although existential concerns and challenges can be observed throughout the illness trajectory, they appear to be paramount during the final stages of cancer. Doka (1993) has written about the unique concerns of living with a life-threatening illness and the needs of dying patients as they reach the end of life.

Questions frequently arise about the existence of God and why, if there *is* a God, did he seemingly abandon someone? As a dying person becomes closer to death, they may reconnect with faith.

Religious and spiritual needs are not synonymous. Hospice professionals attempt to broaden this concept, focusing on the patient's relationship with a higher being, their family, or themselves. Spiritual distress at the end of life creates a crisis for both the dying patient and the family that supports that patient. At times, relationships can become more intense and closely entwined. However, the reverse may be also true; i. e., individuals may grow apart without an attempt to reconcile their differences.

CASE STUDY

> Tony was a 74-year-old retired lawyer who was dying of bladder cancer. He had lost contact with his three children many years ago after he abandoned his family. Although not physically abusive, he had been verbally abusive to his wife and children. While on the hospice program, his primary caregiver was his longtime friend, an old fraternity colleague who knew about Tony's desire to see his adult children and ask for their forgiveness. With the assistance of Tony's hospice social worker and chaplain, a meeting was arranged between Tony and his adult children giving Tony the opportunity to ask for forgiveness.

Frequently, at the end of life, the dying person will reflect back on his or her life, questioning the meaning and significance of that life. Viktor Frankl (1946) described his experiences as a survivor of Auschwitz and maintained that those prisoners who were unable to create meaning psychologically gave up hope and became apathetic, lost faith, and did not survive the concentration camps. Frankl maintained that physical discomfort (pain) and deprivation alone, no matter how extreme, does not cause suffering. The true cause of human suffering, Frankl says, stems from the loss of meaning in one's life. He used his early experiences to illustrate the importance of meaning as a basic drive in human psychology (Breitbart, 2003), as humans seek a sense of meaning or purpose in life as well as in death. We don't have the freedom to prevent death, but we do have the freedom to choose our attitude. Meaning can be found not only in hopes for the future but also in the joys of the past and present.

The crisis surrounding end-of-life care is fertile ground for the importance of rituals. Rituals are always associated with providing a framework for marking significant events in one's life: birth, communion or bar mitzvah, graduation, marriage, and death. Healing rituals around dying can be secular, cultural, or religious. They can provide a meaningful way for families, friends, and the dying patient to communicate in a personal way, perhaps giving voice without actually saying the words.

CASE STUDY

> Brian, a 51-year-old longshoreman dying of prostate cancer orchestrated the making of video tapes for his children and future grandchildren. At the suggestion of his therapist, the tapes were initiated when he enrolled in a home hospice program. Each taping was done at his home (sometimes with his family surrounding him and sometimes alone with the therapist). Concluding the day before he died, Brian's tapes were part life review (reviewing his childhood and teenage years, his marriage, and the "failures" as well as the accomplishments of his life) and part ethical will (focusing on his hopes for his wife and children's future). Ten months after Brian's death, his family organized a "Celebration of His Life." Friends, colleagues, and family members joined to share stories and celebrate the remarkable man he was. Brian's wife made a journal composed of his stories and photographs—distributing the journal to all who attended.

PSYCHOLOGICAL ISSUES AND CONCERNS

Patients with advanced cancers experience many painful and distressing psychiatric and psychological symptoms that may arise from long-standing stressors. These symptoms may be exacerbated by the dying process or they may be new manifestations. Thoughts of suicide, depression, heightened anxiety, panic attacks, and delirium are just some of the overwhelming problems dying patients and their families may confront. There has been an increasing awareness of the benefits in improving one's quality of life and the role of the psychiatrist or psychologist at the end of life (Breitbart & Holland, 1992).

Research has shown that suicidal thoughts frequently surface initially when an individual is first diagnosed with cancer (Hem, Loge, Haldorsen, & Ekeberg, 2004; Allebeck, Bolund, & Ringback, 1989), and tends to recede during the course of the illness only to resurface during the terminal phase (Doka, 2009). The risk of suicide in cancer patients is generally higher than the overall population (Chochinov, Wilson, Enns, & Lander, 1998). Some studies have indicated they are twice as high (Fox, Stanek, Boyd, & Flannery, 1982) and markedly increased for male patients with respiratory cancers (Hem et al., 2004; Allebeck et al., 1989), cancers of the head and neck (Kendal, 2007), and gastrointestinal tumors (Allebeck et al., 1989). A study of 723,810 breast cancer survivors in the United States and Scandinavia found that the risk for suicide was elevated throughout follow-up including for 25 or more years after diagnosis (Schairer et al., 2006). This risk was highest for black women and was increased with the stage of breast cancer.

In one study, 92 terminally ill cancer patients were assessed to identify the prevalence of, and factors contributing to, a desire for hastened death. Researchers determined that the desire for hastened death was not uncommon and that depression and hopelessness were the strongest predictors of desire for hastened death (Breitbart et al., 2000). A study of 200 terminally ill cancer patients in two palliative care inpatient units noted that hopelessness appeared to be a greater clinical marker than depression associated with suicidal ideation (Chochinov et al., 1998). The median survival time from the date of interview to the date of death was 43 days.

In a study of 103 cancer patients enrolled in a home care program, 24 were assessed, followed, and monitored for suicidal ideation (Schachter, Olivieri, Sison, & Farkas, 1993). The presenting psychiatric diagnosis for these 24 patients included major depression (n=7), adjustment disorder with mixed emotional features (n=6), adjustment disorder with depressed mood (n=5), adjustment disorder with anxiety (n=4), organic mood disorder (n=2), and generalized anxiety disorder (n=1). Loss of control and helplessness is perhaps the single most important vulnerability in cancer suicide.

CASE STUDY

> Sandy, a 62-year-old accountant, had been treated for lung cancer. He was divorced, living alone, and had three adult children who lived out of state. When first diagnosed, he tried to electrocute himself while taking a bath. He underwent medical and psychiatric treatment but 1 year after diagnosis, he had a meeting with his oncologist to review his latest scans. At the same time an appointment had been scheduled with his nurse to make a home visit at 9 a.m. the next morning. When the nurse arrived at the scheduled time, it appeared that he was

not at home. She was trying to gain entry into the home when the maid arrived with the key. Upon entrance the nurse found Sandy in bed with his bedside lamp lit, his glasses on, and a book at his side. He was dead and his night table contained an empty bottle of pills.

Individuals who experience a life-threatening illness often feel helpless, forced with the realization that they have lost control over their lives. This loss of control threatens their independence by fostering a dependency on others, which can trigger feelings of being a burden. For individuals who have lived alone, the very thought of having other people in their homes is viewed as intrusive and an invasion of their privacy. They may be able to intellectually acknowledge their need for others, but on an emotional level, their dependency on others is frightening and signifies that death is near.

The need to preserve autonomy is often threatened during the terminal phase. However, we have to be careful of well-meaning family and professional caregivers who may seek to protect the dying patient by making decisions for them. Patients, especially those living alone, have a great deal of difficulty accepting interventions by caring family members or friends. Their loss of independence and the deterioration of their cognitive and physical function highlight their vulnerability and distress.

Anxiety at the end of life escalates and can create turmoil for both the patient and the family. Sometimes patients describe being afraid of pain and the dying process or of what will happen to their loved ones. "I'm so scared." "Why is God punishing me?" "This will go on for a long, long time because my heart is strong." "I'm going to suffer." "If I were older it would have been over already." "I must have done something wrong." "It's not fair." "I'm not ready to give up." "I can't." "How could I just *not be*?"

CASE STUDY

> Sadly, Ethel could not actualize, visualize, or verbalize any meaning in her life. Her past and present psychiatric history so overshadowed her life that she could not focus or find worth in her existence. She was profoundly depressed and anxious yet did not want to be admitted into the hospital inpatient unit: "...underneath it all I'm sad, empty....I wake up crying....This is a difficult time. Intellectually part of me understands many things, but part of me feels, what's all this for? I don't think I can overcome and go on. I'm tired. In all of these years of treatment

and analysis, I'm still the same: dumb old me, and so what? There is no pleasure…If I could get down the stairs I would stand in front of traffic. I want to end this; I don't want to be aware of what's happening; I want to be knocked out. I'm not looking for someone to answer me; I just need to talk" (Schachter, personal conversation, September 5, 1997).

CONCLUSION

Connor (2009) cautions that dying is not a time for intense psychotherapy; it's not a time to unearth new issues. Yet therapeutic alliances and relationships can develop quickly and "transference can occur earlier and more intensely (p. 12). The relationship between the hospice staff (e.g., psychologist, social worker, nurse, chaplain) and the patient and family has the potential to develop quickly and greatly help those at the end of life find peace. Hospice philosophy and care enable clinicians to nurture and develop these relationships helping the patient and family manage all end-of-life concerns: the medical, existential, social, and psychological challenges allowing the patient and family to maintain a sense of equilibrium and peace as they continue to live until they die.

Sherry R. Schachter, PhD, FT, is the director of bereavement services for Calvary Hospital/Hospice where she develops, coordinates, and facilitates educational services for staff and families. She facilitates weekly bereavement groups for bereaved spouses and partners, adults whose parents have died, and parents who have lost children. Dr. Schachter is a recipient of the prestigious Lane Adams Award for Excellence in Cancer Nursing from the American Cancer Society and has worked for over 28 years with dying patients and their family caregivers. In addition, Dr. Schachter has a private practice in New York City and Pennsylvania and also publishes and lectures on issues related to dying, death, and loss. She is the past president of the Association for Death Education and Counseling (ADEC) and a member of the International Work Group on Death, Dying and Bereavement (IWG). Dr. Schachter is the mother of five and grandmother of eight.

References

Allebeck, P., Bolund, C., & Ringback, G. (1989). Increased suicide rate in cancer patients: A cohort study based on the Swedish cancer-environment register. *Journal Clinical Epidemiology, 42*(7), 611–616.

Breitbart, W. (2003). Reframing hope: Meaning-centered care for patients near the end of life: An interview with William Breitbart, MD. *Innovations in End-of-Life Care, 4*(6). Retrieved September 17, 2003 from http://www.edc.org/lastacts

Breitbart, W., & Holland, J. C. (Eds.). (1992). *Psychiatric aspects of symptom management in cancer patients.* Washington, DC: American Psychiatric Press.

Breitbart, W., Rosenfeld, B., Pessin, H., Kaim, M., Funesti-Esch, J., Galietta, M., et al. (2000). Depression, hopelessness, and desire for hastened death in terminally ill patients with cancer. *JAMA, 284*, 2907–2911.

Chochinov, H. M., Wilson, K. G., Enns, M., & Lander, S. (1998, August). Depression, hopelessness, and suicidal ideation in the terminally ill. *Psychosomatics, 39*(4), 366–370.

Christakis, N. A. (1994, June). Timing of referral of terminally ill patients to an outpatient hospice. *Journal of General Internal Medicine, 9*, 314–320.

Connor, S. (2009). *Hospice and palliative care: The essential guide.* New York: Routledge.

Doka, K. J. (1993). *Living with a life-threatening illness.* New York: Lexington Books.

Doka, K. J. (2009). *Counseling individuals with life-threatening illness.* New York: Springer.

Dunn, H. (n.d.). *Hard choices for loving people.* Retrieved June 24, 2009 from http://www.hospicenet.org/html/choices-pr.html

Fox, B. H., Stanek, E. J., Boyd, S. C., & Flannery, J. T. (1982). Suicide rates among cancer patients in Connecticut. *Journal Chronic Diseases, 35*(2), 89–100.

Frankl, V. E. (1946). *Man's search for meaning.* New York: Simon & Schuster. (Original translation by Beacon Press in 1959).

Friedrichsen, M. J., & Strang, P. M. (2003). Doctors' strategies when breaking bad news to terminally ill patients. *Journal of Palliative Medicine, 6*(4), 565–574.

Hem, E., Loge, J. H., Haldorsen, T., & Ekeberg, D. (2004). Suicide risk in cancer patients from 1960 to 1999. Presented at the 25th European Conference on Psychosomatic Research, Berlin, Germany, June 23–26.

Kendal, W. S. (2007). Suicide and cancer: A gender-comparative study. *Annals of Oncology, 18*(2), 381–387.

Lee, S. J., Fairclough, D., Antin, J. H., & Woods, J. C. (2001). Discrepancies between patient and physician estimates for the success of stem cell transplantation. *JAMA, 285*(5), 1034–1038.

Mackillop, W. J., & Quirt, C. F. (1997). Measuring the accuracy of prognostic judgments in oncology. *Journal of Clinical Epidemiology, 50*(1), 21–29.

Miyaji, N. (1993). The power of compassion: Truth-telling among American doctors in the care of dying patients. *Social Science and Medicine, 36,* 249–264.

Righetti, A., & Giorgio, G. (1994). Factors influencing the communication of the diagnosis to patients who have cancer. *Journal of Cancer Education, 9,* 42–45.

Schachter, S. R. (September 5, 1997). Personal conversation.

Schachter, S. R. (1999). The experience of living with a life-threatening illness: A phenomenological study of dying cancer patients and their family caregivers. Unpublished dissertation. Cincinnati, OH: Union Institute University.

Schachter, S. R. (2009). Cancer patients facing death. In M. K. Bartalos (Ed.), *Speaking of death: America's new sense of mortality* (pp. 42–77). Westport, CT: Praeger Publishers.

Schachter, S. R., & Coyle, N. (1998). Palliative home care—impact on families. In J. C. Holland (Ed.), *Psycho-Oncology* (pp. 1004–1015). New York: Oxford University Press.

Schachter, S. R., Olivieri, A. P., Sison, A. C., & Farkas, C. G. (1993, October 2). Suicidal ideation in patients with advanced disease managed in a psychiatry home care program. Presented at the Psycho Oncology V: Psychosocial factors in cancer risk and survival. New York City.

Schairer, C., Brown, L. M., Chen, B. E., Howard, R., Lynch, C. F., Hall, et al. (2006). Brief communication: Suicide after breast cancer: An international population-based study of 723,810 women. *Journal of the National Cancer Institute, 98*(19), 1416–1419.

SUPPORT Principal Investigators. (1995). A controlled trial to improve care for seriously ill hospitalized patients: The study to understand prognoses and preferences for outcomes and risks of treatments (SUPPORT). *JAMA, 274*(20), 1591–1598.

United States Department of Health and Human Services. (2000). *Medicare Hospice Benefits* (CMS Publication No. 02154). Retrieved August 26, 2008 from http://www.medicare.gov/publications/Pubs/pdf/02154.pdf

Weeks, J. C., Cook, E. F., O'Day, S. J., Peterson, L. M., Wenger, N., Reding, D., et al. (1998). Relationship between cancer patients' predictions of prognosis and their treatment preferences. *JAMA, 279*(21), 1709–1714.

Winterling, J., Wasteson, E., Glimelius, B., Sjoden, P. O., & Nordin, K. (2004). Substantial changes in life. *Cancer Nursing, 27*(5), 381–388.

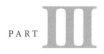

Psychosocial Aspects of Cancer Care

I f there is one lesson to be learned from hospice, it is that treating any disease, especially one as complex as cancer, necessitates holistic care. We cannot afford to treat only the disease; rather, we must treat the whole person. Cancer in particular raises a host of spiritual and psychosocial issues. *Why did I receive the disease? Why now?* These questions, asked for any disease, are ultimately spiritual concerns. Lifestyle factors such as substance abuse or alcohol and tobacco use may be a factor in diseases such as lung or liver cancers, leading to themes of guilt, blame, and punishment.

Moreover, there are psychological and spiritual residues even in recovery. Patients may cope with ongoing anxiety over the possibility of recurrence. Persons may have to reconstruct their identities if they are coping with disfigurement or amputations. Mastectomies, impotency, or erectile dysfunction may be a consequence of cancer care, challenging gender identity.

Krajewski, Costanzo, LoConte, and LoConte begin this section with a chapter on the issue of guilt in cancer patients. They affirm that guilt can be a significant aspect of cancer care that goes beyond simply acknowledging risk factors such as tobacco use. Cancer patients may feel guilt over a range of factors including neglecting appropriate cancer screening tests, delaying diagnosis, or even living a stressful lifestyle. At the end of life, patients may feel that they did not fight hard enough. The authors recognize that guilt can have both positive and negative effects. Guilt can be associated with anxiety and depression. However, it also can be a motivational spur, causing patients to be more vigilant in monitoring the disease and treatment, and to avoid self-destructive behaviors. Krajewski, Costanzo, LoConte, and LoConte's chapter reminds clinicians of two critical factors. First, they need to explore patients' perspectives on both cancer causation and treatment. Second, they need to be attentive to the patient's guilt issues and explore the ways that the patient is coping with that loss.

Marianne Walsh notes the many distinct issues that are experienced by children and adolescents with cancer. She notes that when a child or adolescent experiences cancer, it challenges the parents' assumptive world as we naturally assume that our children will outlive us. Walsh reaffirms the importance of communication and the roles that expressive therapies can have in facilitating communication and helping children and adolescents cope with the disease.

Many of Walsh's comments are validated in Mary Martin's personal perspective on her infant's death from a rare form of brain cancer. Martin illustrates the very difficult issue of deciding, especially with a child, when care becomes palliative.

Neil Thompson offers a chapter on the role of gender in cancer. Thompson describes the multiple ways that cancer and gender interact. At the most obvious level, certain forms of cancer, such as cervical or prostate, are only found in one gender. In other cases, gender expectations can stigmatize victims. For example, men can have breast cancer. For such men, the association between breast cancer and womanhood can be isolating. Thompson's chapter explores the many ways that gender can influence responses to the disease as well as ways that cancer can challenge gender identity. He reminds health professionals that the implications of the disease for gender cannot be overlooked.

Thompson's piece also reinforces the need to view the larger social context in responding to cancer. While Thompson focuses on gender, there are significant disparities in cancer morbidity based on race, ethnicity, and social class. Gross, Smith, Wolf, and Andersen (2008), in reviewing the decade between 1992 and 2002, note that even with Medicare and other programs, such disparities still exist. Their research echoes a theme of this book. Only comprehensive, culturally appropriate programs that consider the social surroundings and address the patient's sense of stigma, anxieties, and personal perspective on cancer causation and treatment are likely to mitigate these disparities.

REFERENCE

Gross, C. P., Smith, B. D., Wolf, E., & Andersen, M. (2008). Racial disparities in cancer therapy: Did the gap narrow between 1992 and 2002? *Cancer*, *112*(4), 900–908.

CHAPTER 10

Guilt and Self-Blame: Coping with Cancer Causation

Kenneth A. Krajewski, Erin S. Costanzo, Matthew D. LoConte, and Noelle K. LoConte

G uilt and self-blame in cancer patients and their caregivers is an important psychological issue that may be inadequately addressed in the healthcare setting. Over a half century ago, a study conducted at the Massachusetts General Hospital reviewed feelings of guilt and their effect on the lives of cancer patients and caregivers (Abrams & Finesinger, 1953). The study called on physicians, nurses, and social workers to help alleviate feelings of guilt in order to improve the mental health of cancer patients with hopes of bringing better rehabilitation. However, research on guilt and self-blame in the setting of cancer remains an understudied area. To summarize the overall findings in the current literature, guilt and self-blame are typically associated with poorer psychological adjustment (such as higher levels of depression or anxiety), but can also lead to positive adjustment, or a motivation to change behavior. For example, a study led by Bulman and Wortman (1977) with paralyzed accident victims suggests that self-blame can be viewed as an internal cause and be perceived as controllable and therefore changeable.

A review of current literature was performed regarding patients' beliefs about the causes of their cancer and self-blame attributions, and their relation to the psychological adjustment of cancer patients and their caretakers. Results will be discussed by cancer type, which reflects the organization of many current studies.

BREAST CANCER AND DISTRESS

Breast cancer is the cancer most broadly studied for the impact of self-blame and psychological adjustment. Competing theories exist regarding psychological adjustment in breast cancer patients with self-blame attributions (Bennett, Compas, Beckjord, & Glinder, 2005; Glinder & Compas, 1999; Lavery & Clarke, 1996). It has been argued that self-blame attributions can cause psychological distress and poorer adjustment, including symptoms of depression. Another view is that self-blame can lead to positive adjustment, as earlier described with paralysis victims (Bulman & Wortman, 1977) and in subsequent studies of breast cancer survivors (Stewart et al., 2001; Rabin & Pinto, 2006).

A recent study examined behavioral and characterological self-blame attributions as well as psychological distress in newly diagnosed breast cancer patients (Bennett et al., 2005). Behavioral self-blame is defined as blame focused on behavior that a person engages in such as smoking cigarettes. Characterological self-blame is directed at stable aspects of character and personality, for example perceiving that one has a history of bad luck. The authors hypothesized that both forms of self-blame attributions would create psychological distress shortly following diagnosis. It was also hypothesized that over time, characterological self-blame would be associated with distress, whereas behavioral self-blame allows control and would protect against distress. The study validated that both forms of self-blame in patients with newly diagnosed breast cancer experienced psychological distress at 4 months postdiagnosis. Characterological self-blame at 7 and 12 months postdiagnosis was associated with distress—more so for depression than anxiety. The study was unable to validate that only characterological self-blame predicted a trend of distress at 7 and 12 months as psychological distress was also seen in patients with behavioral self-blame. Similar results have been found in other studies (Malcarne, Compas, Epping-Jordan, & Howell, 1995).

The results of this set of studies suggest that attributions of self-blame in cancer patients may adversely affect psychological adjustment and this is consistent with a recent review (Friedman et al., 2007), which found that self-blame among cancer patients was related to greater mood disturbance and a poorer quality of life. In contrast, self-forgiveness can enhance psychological well-being and protect against cancer-related distress. Specifically, Romero et al. (2005) studied 81 breast cancer patients in a medical oncology clinic and found self-forgiveness and spirituality were unique predictors of less mood disturbance and better quality of life. Another study found that those who had a more self-forgiving nature were less likely to blame themselves for breast cancer and were better adjusted to their cancer. Additional studies show that women who believed that lifestyle factors (such as diet) contributed to their cancer were more likely to make positive changes in these areas after their cancer was diagnosed (Costanzo, Lutgendorf, Mattes, & Trehan, 2006; Rabin & Pinto, 2006).

GYNECOLOGICAL CANCER

In this category, cancer survivors' perceived factors about the causes of cancer were only partially consistent with current scientific knowledge (Wold, Byers, Crane, & Ahnen 2005; Costanzo, Lutgendorf, Bradley, Rose, & Anderson, 2005). Endometrial and cervical cancer patients' most commonly reported factors causing their cancer were genetics/heredity, stress, and God's will (see Table 1) (Costanzo et al., 2005).

TABLE 1. Significantly Different Mean Scores of Perceived Cancer-Related Stigma Items at Enrollment

Statement	Non-small cell lung cancer (mean score)*	Comparison [breast and prostate] (mean score)*	p-value
I am ashamed I got my type of cancer.	1.79	1.15	<0.001
My family feels ashamed of my type of cancer.	1.52	1.23	<0.05
I am embarrassed to tell people my type of cancer.	1.68	1.32	<0.05
My behavior contributed to my type of cancer.	2.66	1.69	<0.001

* Scored from 1 to 5, with 1 meaning "strongly agree" and 5 meaning "strongly disagree" (LoConte et al., 1998).

Stress ranked second, with 46% of patients rating it to be somewhat to very important to the development of their cancer. Although the media may also portray this belief, Costanzo et al. reported that the scientific literature is inconclusive (2005). Patients underestimated hormonal factors (as it was ranked fourth) for both types of cancer. The majority of patients did not rank tobacco, lifestyle, or diet as important causes of cancer. Cervical cancer survivors overlooked the importance of multiple sexual partners, tobacco, early intercourse, and healthy diet including vitamins A and C. Additional endometrial cancer risk factors underrated were high-fat diet, obesity, and physical exercise.

Personal theories may develop on how to control one's cancer and prevent recurrence. Gynecological cancer patients rated medical checkups or screenings followed by a positive attitude, prayer, and diet as the top factors in preventing recurrence (Costanzo et al., 2005). Healthy lifestyle, diet, and exercise are known risk factors for reducing gynecological cancer and they fell toward the middle of the survey results. In contrast from perceived cancer causation, God's will and chance were rated toward the end of the list of factors for recurrence. Costanzo et al. noted that perhaps the most interesting finding in preventing cancer recurrence was that 94% of gynecological cancer survivors rated a positive attitude as somewhat to very important (2005). The authors state that there is slightly more evidence in the literature that a positive attitude and "fighting spirit" are associated with a reduced risk of cancer recurrence and better survival. However, it is noted that data are still conflicting and far from compelling.

This study further examined the complex relationships between patients' attributions and both their psychological adjustment and the behavioral accommodations they make following cancer treatment. The authors found that a stronger belief that one's cancer was caused by controllable factors was linked to increased anxiety and depressive symptomatology, but also to more positive health practices (Costanzo et al., 2005). Specifically, gynecological patients who made positive health behavior changes following their diagnosis, including obtaining regular cancer screening, were more likely to attribute their cancer to controllable causes such as stress and unhealthy lifestyle (ibid.). Compared to women who were not practicing positive health behaviors, these women were also more likely to believe diet, stress reduction, exercise, and medical screenings could prevent recurrence. Follow-up analyses clarified that the belief that controllable factors such as an unhealthy lifestyle may contribute to cause or recurrence was associated with greater distress only in women who failed to improve their health habits after their diagnosis. Conversely, in women who made positive changes to their health behaviors, attributing cancer to controllable factors did not cause additional anxiety or depression.

Figure 1 illustrates this interaction for women who made positive changes in their diet versus those who did not. Thus, the cancer attributions that focus on personal control may be associated with greater distress, but engaging in behavior thought to prevent cancer recurrence reduces this distress (Costanzo et al., 2005).

FIGURE 1: Interaction between Attributing Cancer to an Unhealthy Lifestyle and Dietary Change in Predicting Anxiety

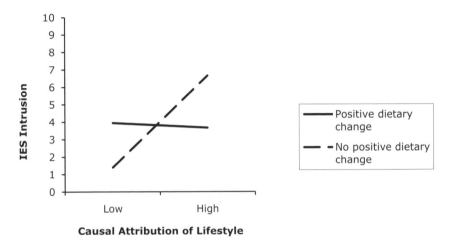

Note. High and low points represent scores one standard deviation above and below the mean on lifestyle attribution. Reprinted with permission from Wolters Kluwer Health.

LUNG CANCER AND PERCEIVED RISK AMONG SMOKERS

It is widely known among healthcare providers that of all modifiable risk factors, smoking causes the most preventable deaths from cardiovascular disease and cancer and the smoking/lung cancer causation link is among the strongest lifestyle-related risks in oncology (Ayanian & Cleary, 1999). Thus, lung cancer patients face the most stigma for their cancer. However, not all smokers perceive their risk to be as high. For example, a study in conjunction with Harvard Medical School looked at cigarette smokers' perceived risk of cancer and heart disease (ibid). Over 3000 participants age 25 to 74 were surveyed and of that population, 24.3% were current smokers. Interestingly, smokers did not perceive their own personal risk of disease from tobacco use to be very high. Only 29% of current smokers thought they were at higher than average risk for a myocardial infarction and 40% thought they had increased risk of cancer. Additionally, only 49% of heavy smokers (over 40 cigarettes daily) reported having higher than average risk for cancer. The authors noted this is consistent with prior studies where smokers fail to recognize their personal risk for cardiovascular events and cancer.

A study of recently diagnosed lung cancer patients undergoing radiation or chemotherapy found that all 52 participants had a smoking history and 8% reported feelings of guilt (Ginsburg, Quirt, Ginsburg, & MacKillop, 1995). Thirteen percent used terms like "angry," "mad," and "cheated," while the study stated denial was apparent in 15%. One participant reported he had "brought this on [himself] because of [his] lifestyle of drinking and smoking." Another patient wondered what he had done "to end up like this" and how his lung cancer was affected by smoking, drinking, and painting cars without a mask. Other studies have shown that lung cancer patients frequently do not perceive their cancer as being related to their prior smoking, though this is not a universal finding (Bertero, Vanhanen, & Appelin, 2008; Mumma & McCorkle, 1983). Other studies have shown that believing one caused one's cancer led to a strong perception of control over the cancer (Berckman & Austin, 1993).

COMPARISON OF NON-SMALL-CELL LUNG CANCER TO OTHER CANCERS

A recent study published in the *British Medical Journal* interviewed a diverse group (i.e., age, race, and gender) of patients with lung cancer to explore their perceptions and experienced stigma (Chapple, Ziebland, & McPherson, 2004). The study was unique in its format using interviews with open-ended questions and highlighting interesting narratives from participants. Regardless of whether patients had a smoking history, they felt particularly stigmatized compared to other cancers because the disease was so strongly associated with smoking and because lung cancer patients can die in an unpleasant way. The stigma, both "felt" and "enacted," can affect interactions with family, friends, and even with physicians. Patients reported that acquaintances they have known for years would cross the street to avoid contact with them because they did not know what to say. Another patient reported her daughter had not telephoned because she felt "dirtied" by her contact with cancer. Similar findings have been reported in other studies.

The British study discussed lung cancer patients' personal views on a variety of topics including political aspects and tobacco companies. Participants noted the substantial disparity in research funding and screening programs between lung and other types of cancer such as breast cancer. Participants said this may be related to the fact that lung cancer is smoking related and "self-inflicted." A few patients resist personal responsibility for smoking and "victim blaming." One participant states it is the "tobacco manufacturers' fault for putting the carcinogens in in the first place." Many others, particularly support group members, cited other potential causes of their cancer including diesel fumes, carbon monoxide, spray paint, asbestos, pollution, stress, diet, and bereavement.

A 2007 study examined guilt and shame in patients with non-small-cell lung cancer (NSCLC) to a comparison group with cancers largely unrelated to lifestyle choices (breast and prostate cancer) (Else-Quest, LoConte, Schiller, & Hyde, 2008; LoConte, Else-Quest, Eickhoff, Hyde, & Schiller, 2008). The study was conducted to determine if lung cancer patients had more guilt and shame as a result of previous smoking. Participants had stage IV NSCLC, breast cancer, and prostate cancer and were surveyed three times (at enrollment, 2 months, and 6 months). In this study, 29.5% of patients with NSCLC and 10.5% of the comparison group thought their past behaviors contributed to their cancer. The most frequent response from all surveyed members to an open ended "What do you believe caused your cancer?" was "I don't know." Breast and prostate cancer patients were more likely than lung cancer patients to report uncertainty in the etiology of their cancer. The second most common response was smoking, followed by environmental causes such as pollution and asbestos. Heredity was also reported, followed by a minority reporting stress, lifestyle factors (e.g., diet and exercise), hormone therapy, second-hand smoke, and Agent Orange exposure.

Among patients with lung cancer, 80.2% were previous smokers, 11.5% were current smokers, and 8.3% reported having never smoked. The comparison group of breast and prostate cancer patients consisted of 67.1% previous or current smokers and 32.9% who had never smoked. Previous and current smokers with lung cancer had higher mean guilt and shame scores than nonsmokers. Greater guilt and shame was also seen in breast and prostate cancer patients with a smoking history. The study found smoking status, regardless of cancer type, was significantly associated with feelings of guilt and shame.

A study with the same sample found that in addition to smoking status, type of cancer also predicted feelings of guilt and shame. Specifically, LoConte et al. developed the Perceived Cancer-Related Stigma (PCRS) scale to assess self-blame, guilt, and embarrassment related to cancer (2008). This is a composite score that assesses the degree to which patients blame themselves or their behavior for their cancer. In addition, the State Shame and Guilt Scale (SSGS) was used to assess current levels of generalized guilt and shame. Patients with NSCLC were significantly more likely to agree with the PCRS items including "I am ashamed I got my type of cancer," "My family feels ashamed of my type of cancer," "I am embarrassed to tell people my type of cancer," and "My behavior contributed to my type of cancer." However, neither NSCLC patients nor the comparison group agreed with "I deserve my type of cancer" and "People judge me for my type of cancer" (see Table 1).

HEAD AND NECK CANCERS

Head and neck cancers are also strongly related to prior smoking and alcohol intake. Patients who continue to smoke are more likely to have a recurrence of their cancer after primary treatment. Investigators have determined that perceived control over cancer and self-blame for one's cancer interact to determine likelihood of continuing to smoke after a diagnosis of head and neck cancer (Christensen et al., 1999). More specifically, among patients who did not believe that their cancer was caused by past behaviors, only those who perceived a high level of control over their cancer quit smoking. Additional relationships were also found to exist. For example, among patients who did feel past behavior contributed to their cancer, only those who felt they had control over their cancer situation quit smoking after being diagnosed with cancer.

FAMILY CAREGIVERS AND GUILT

A 2008 study funded by the American Cancer Society reviewed caregiver guilt as a key emotional phenomenon (Spillers, Wellisch, Youngmee, Matthews, & Baker, 2008). The study reports being the first of its kind to explore cancer caregiver stress factors associated with caregiver guilt and, in addition, the association of caregivers' guilt with their adjustment outcomes. The American Cancer Society's Quality of Life Survey for Caregivers is a 5-year longitudinal study that has produced the article titled "Family Caregivers and Guilt in the Context of Cancer Care" (ibid.). Caregiver was defined as an unpaid family member or close friend providing care to the cancer survivor. A Caregiver Guilt

Scale, composed of statements for caregivers to rate based on personal feelings when caring for another person, was created and validated by 12 experts. The study identified that an employed, younger adult offspring was more likely to experience caregiver guilt as they had to balance employment demands and their own family life (ibid.). This finding was consistent with a 2003 study that investigated caregivers of breast cancer hospice patients (Lobchuk, Murdoch, McClement, & McPherson, 2008). Higher caregiver guilt was associated with a busy schedule and a loved one whose overall health was poor (Spillers et al., 2008). Patients with declining or poor health may require additional care, which means more time and interruptions in the caregiver's personal schedule. The researchers state: "These findings may reflect the caregiver's feeling of being overwhelmed and realizing little or no satisfaction in providing care for a person who cannot seem to improve regardless of the caregiver's efforts." Under these circumstances, the caregiver is especially susceptible to guilt.

Caregiver guilt was inversely related to their perceived competence. The study acknowledges family caregivers have a strong sense of commitment to providing exceptional care. Personal feelings of incompetency may lead to guilt and inadequacy and ultimately a sense of failed obligation. Guilt may reach an apex when caring for the dying cancer patient as no task, regardless of performance and competency, seems to improve quantity or quality of life.

An important finding by Spillers et al. was a strong relationship between caregivers' guilt and their adjustment outcomes for psychological distress and mental, social, and physical functioning. Mental and social functioning was defined by levels of social adjustment including vitality, mental health, and emotional adjustment to social roles. The authors reported burdened caregivers were more likely to withdraw socially. Caregiver guilt seemed to compromise social adjustment, which may lead to social withdrawal and role strain. Increased caregiver guilt appeared to increase psychological distress and diminish physical functioning (e.g., increased somatic complaints).

CLOSING

Personal beliefs about an individual's medical condition may influence both health behaviors and psychological distress. Generally, cancer attribution and self-blame is related to greater distress, but possibly only among patients who do not then make efforts to change the behavior or the factor that they believe caused their cancer. Additionally, characterological self-blame seems to have a more adverse effect on psychological adjustment than behavioral self-blame, perhaps because behavioral self-blame may enhance feelings of control.

Finally, controllable attributions may also be related to more positive health practices, and self-forgiveness can protect against cancer-related distress. Self-blame, particularly behavioral self-blame, may enhance feelings of control. Greater perceived control is associated with fewer depressive symptoms and better adjustment.

Patients should be informed about known risk factors for cancer causation to reduce their risk of recurrence and educate the general population. Healthcare professionals need to recognize and discuss feelings of guilt or shame associated with a patient's diagnosis and intervene to ease anxiety and symptoms of depression. Cancer patients and caregivers should address "What role has the illness taken on your relationship?" and "How are you handling the changes imposed by the cancer on your social life?" The findings of the studies also have several implications for psychosocial or behavioral interventions: Teaching self-forgiveness, or helping patients to make positive changes in health practices, would appear to alleviate distress related to self-blame. Additional research is needed in a variety of areas regarding blame, guilt, and coping among cancer patients and caregivers for improved knowledge and understanding to better meet their psychological needs.

Dr. Krajewski is an internal medicine resident at the University of Wisconsin. Dr. Costanzo is an assistant professor at the UW School of Medicine and Public Health and a cancer psychologist at the UW Paul Carbone Comprehensive Cancer Center. Dr. Matt LoConte is a clinical assistant professor of medicine at UW, the director of palliative care at the William S. Middleton Memorial VA Hospital in Madison, Wisconsin, and medical director at Hospice Care, Inc. in Fitchburg, Wisconsin. Dr. Noelle LoConte is assistant professor of medicine at the UW School of Medicine and Public Health, and is a medical oncologist specializing in geriatric and gastrointestinal oncology.

REFERENCES

Abrams, R. D., & Finesinger, J. E. (1953). Guilt reactions in patients with cancer. *Cancer, 6*, 474–482.

Ayanian, J. Z., & Cleary, P. D. (1999). Perceived risks of heart disease and cancer among cigarette smokers. *JAMA, 281*, 1019–1021.

Bennett, K. K., Compas, B. E., Beckjord, E., & Glinder, J. G. (2005). Self-blame and distress among women with newly diagnosed breast cancer. *Journal of Behavioral Medicine, 28*(4), 313–323.

Berckman, K. L., & Austin, J. K. (1993). Causal attribution, perceived control, and adjustment in patients with lung cancer. *Oncology Nursing Forum, 20,* 23–30.

Bertero, C., Vanhanen, M., & Appelin, G. (2008). Receiving a diagnosis of inoperable lung cancer: Patients' perspectives of how it affects their life situation and quality of life. *Acta Oncologica, 47,* 862–869.

Bulman, R. J., & Wortman, C. B. (1977). Attributions of blame and coping in the "real world": Severe accident victims react to their lot. *Journal of Personality and Social Psychology, 35,* 351–363.

Chapple, A., Ziebland, S., & McPherson, A. (2004). Stigma, shame, and blame experienced by patients with lung cancer: Qualitative study. *British Medical Journal, 328,* 1470–1474.

Christensen, A. J., Moran, P. J., Ehlers, S. L., Raichle, K., Karnell, L., & Funk, G. (1999). Smoking and drinking behavior in patients with head and neck cancer: Effects of behavioral self-blame and perceived control. *Journal of Behavioral Medicine, 22,* 407–418.

Costanzo, E. S., Lutgendorf, S. K., Bradley, S. L., Rose, S. L., & Anderson, B. (2005). Cancer attributions, distress, and health practices among gynecologic cancer survivors. *Psychosomatic Medicine, 67,* 972–980.

Costanzo, E. S., Lutgendorf, S. K., Mattes, M. L., & Trehan, S. (2006). Illness perceptions and post-treatment distress and behavior changes among women with breast cancer. *Psychosomatic Medicine, 63,* A-45.

Else-Quest, N. M., LoConte, N. K., Schiller, J. H., & Hyde, J. S. (2008). Perceived stigma, self-blame, and adjustment among lung, breast and prostate cancer patients. *Psychology and Health, 1,* 16.

Friedman, L. C., Romero, C., Elledge, R., Chang, J., Kalidas, M., Dulay, M. F., et al. (2007). Attribution of blame, self-forgiving attitude and psychological adjustment in women with breast cancer. *Journal of Behavioral Medicine, 30,* 351–357.

Ginsburg, M. L., Quirt, C., Ginsburg, A. D., & MacKillop, W. J. (1995). Psychiatric illness and psychosocial concerns of patients with newly diagnosed lung cancer. *Canadian Medical Association Journal, 152*(5), 701–708.

Glinder, J. G., & Compas, B. E. (1999). Self-blame attributions in women with newly diagnosed breast cancer: A prospective study of psychological adjustment. *Health Psychology, 18,* 475–481.

Lavery, J. F., & Clarke, V. A. (1996). Causal attributions, coping strategies, and adjustment to breast cancer. *Cancer Nursing, 19,* 20–28.

Lobchuk, M. M., Murdoch, T., McClement, S. E., & McPherson, C. (2008). A dyadic affair: Who is to blame for causing and controlling the patient's lung cancer? *Cancer Nursing, 31*(6), 435–443.

LoConte, N. K., Else-Quest, N. M., Eickhoff, J., Hyde, J., & Schiller, J. H. (2008). Assessment of guilt and shame in patients with non-small-cell lung cancer compared with patients with breast and prostate cancer. *Clinical Lung Cancer, 9*(3), 171–178.

Malcarne, V. L., Compas, B. E., Epping-Jordan, J. E., & Howell, D. C. (1995). Cognitive factors in adjustment to cancer: Attributions of self-blame and perceptions of control. *Journal of Behavioral Medicine, 18,* 401–417.

Mumma, C., & McCorkle, R. (1983). Causal attribution and life-threatening disease. *International Journal of Psychiatry in Medicine, 12,* 311–319.

Rabin, C., & Pinto, B. (2006). Cancer-related beliefs and health behavior change among breast cancer survivors and their first-degree relatives. *Psychooncology, 15,* 701–712.

Romero, C., Friedman, L. C., Kalidas, M., Elledge, R., Chang, J., & Liscum, K. R. (2005). Self-forgiveness, spirituality, and psychological adjustment in women with breast cancer. *Journal of Behavioral Medicine, 29*(1), 29–36.

Spillers, R. L., Wellisch, D. K., Youngmee, K., Matthews, B. A., & Baker, F. (2008). Family caregivers and guilt in the context of cancer care. *Psychosomatics, 49,* 511–519.

Stewart, D. E., Cheung, A. M., Duff, S., Wong, F., McQuestion, M., Cheng, T., et al. (2001). Attributions of cause and recurrence in long-term breast cancer survivors. *Psychooncology, 10*(2), 179–183.

Wold, K. S., Byers, T., Crane, L. A., & Ahnen, D. (2005). What do cancer survivors believe causes cancer? *Cancer Cause Control, 16,* 115–123.

Cancer in Children and Adolescents: Psychosocial Dimensions

Marianne Walsh

C ancer is the major cause of death by disease in children between the ages of 1 and 14. The National Cancer Institute estimates that in the United States, more than 8,500 children less than 15 years of age are diagnosed each year with cancer (Ries et al., 2004). Leukemias, lymphomas, and central and sympathetic nervous system tumors are responsible for the most cancer deaths in this age group. Soft tissue, bone, and kidney cancers were also common. Trends in cancer deaths for adolescents ages 15 to 19 were led by brain and ONS (other nervous system), leukemia, bones and joints, soft tissue, and non-Hodgkin's lymphoma (ibid.).

In our assumptive world, we expect to outlive our children. Sadly, that is not always the case and unfortunately, instead of our children burying us, we bury our children. Coping with a fatal illness of a child is one of the most stressful events encountered by families. The experience is an emotional roller coaster of dramatic highs and lows, disappointments of yesterday and hope for the future. During this demanding journey, a time comes when curative treatment stops and hope for a cure is transformed into hope for a pain-free death. Cure-oriented treatment must now interface with symptom-oriented care (Hadlock, 1985; Levy, 1985). This transition from curative to palliative care for the terminal child, however, is a difficult and challenging decision for parents. Hinds et al. (1997) report that end-of-life decision making is the most difficult treatment-related decision that parents encounter during their child's cancer experience. We will explore the stressors felt by the child and his or her parents as the disease evolves and the course of psychosocial support for the individuals involved. One parent of a 19-year-old adolescent told me that signing the do-not-resuscitate order 1 week before her daughter's death was the defining moment for her. "It prepared me to say it is okay."

Treatment protocols for cancer are long and arduous, accompanied by many predictable and unpredictable side effects. The treatment is often worse than the disease for many children and adolescents. A child or adolescent's emotions are deep, complex, and can often run rampant; they are scared and may feel compromised. A 15-year-old girl told me that she felt her body was betraying her and allowing some poison (cancer) to grow inside her. Children suffering with cancer feel dramatically powerless as curative treatment continues and invasive procedures are performed on their fragile bodies over which they have no control.

Support staff such as social workers, child life specialists, creative art therapists, and the medical personnel play a significant role in meeting the psychosocial needs of the child and adolescent living with cancer. These services include emotional, social, and psychological support for families and patients to cope with the enormous strains the disease places on them. Barbara Sourkes (1992) writes about the intimacy of the therapeutic relationship in the medical environment in *Countertransference in Psychotherapy with Children and Adolescents:*

> Exposure to suffering is a given in the daily routine of the therapists who consult at a medical center. To an important extent, the therapist's credibility with the seriously ill child is based on his or her ability to tolerate these physical aspects. A child gains a sense of safety in understanding painful procedures if he or she knows that the therapist can at least bear witness to them.

Children start to feel empowered again when they are provided with choices that many of the creative modalities offer. They then have the freedom to choose—to become involved or not participate. In their unique world of disorder and unfamiliarity, they have once again found control. Psychological safety is as important as physical protection, for children's feelings need the same kind of respect and concern as their bodies (Rubin, 1984). Tracy Councill believes that "a supportive, client-centered, and at times non-verbal approach can help the patient both express troubling feelings and regain some sense of bodily integrity and self-worth" (1993).

Children who cannot communicate their angst and fears verbally or through writing convey their feelings through the art process. Art is a natural modality of expression for children whether it is drawing, painting, collage, or clay. Children find it easier to communicate, especially those things they will not or cannot share verbally, through drawing (Bertoia, 1993). One month before dying, Eliza, a 7-year-old female hospice patient whose mother had died 3 years earlier, began to draw a collection of drawings representing being reunited with her mother in heaven. Although bald from chemotherapy, the pictures portrayed Eliza with a full head of long hair walking with her mother who was not ambulatory months before her death. The poignant drawings communicated an awareness of her imminent death and a hope of being reconnected with her mother.

The arts have the healing powers to which children can easily relate. Robert Coles reflects on the drawings of a 10-year-old girl sick with leukemia: "Her drawings told much about the taciturn child, fighting that ultimate terror (death) we all must face, sooner or later, and yet able to evoke with crayons exactly what she was experiencing. Hers was an articulate eloquence—that of visual representation. Put differently, she knew how to put into her drawings a mix of the aesthetic, cognitive, and emotional" (1992). Art truly sustains the child when they are confronted with the prospect of death.

In a palliative care paradigm, a discussion should be had with the patient's parents about communicating about death with the child. Children are aware that they are dying and do sense the overwhelming stress of their parents when death is imminent. They may feel alone and isolated if they are not provided with an opportunity to talk openly about their illness and death (Faulkner, 1997; Whittam, 1993). Young children often present these feelings of death awareness indirectly. These signs usually include heightened separation anxiety, fears that something could happen to the parents or other family members, nightmares, tearfulness, anger issues, noncooperative behaviors, and changes in eating patterns (Sourkes, 1992). The adolescent on the other hand manifests noncommunicative reactions with rage, focus on issues concerning sexuality and appearance, and mindfulness to time (ibid.). Tina, a 19-year-old palliative care patient, impressed upon her mother a day before lapsing into a coma a sense of urgency to have her core group of friends visit. While Tina was surrounded by friends at her bedside, the next day, she held her best friend's hand and took her last breath.

The literature supports the strong belief among professionals that children and adolescents should be provided with honest information regarding their illness and the treatment plan. Trust is a major component in the sick child's life, and maintaining open communication is a path to preserve and sustain that key component. Exploring information with a child at the onset of the illness will establish trust with the child that he or she will be told the truth during the course of the disease (Beale, Baile, & Aaron, 2005). To keep information from a child is both futile and harmful (Doka, 1995). Psychosocial interventions at the end of life promote communication, foster relationships, and deter potential problems. The trained pediatric professional will offer interventions that are age-appropriate with a focus on the child's cognitive and emotional stages of development (Faulkner, 1993).

Often in the child's course of treatment, the question of who tells the child about dying is discussed. While the child remains in the hospital environment, the parents, medical staff, psychosocial staff, and spiritual provider are included in the process. If the child is in the home receiving services from the palliative and hospice team, they include but are not limited to a nurse, social worker, home health aide, and spiritual provider, as well as the parents and family members. As the child's pain and medical decisions are discussed, so is the issue of dying. Opportunities to explore death-related questions present themselves early in a child's cancer journey. Hence, it is critical that all professionals involved with the dying child are aware of the psychosocial care plan. Beale et al. (2005) provide a "6 Es" strategy as a guideline for communicating with the child and family:

1. *Establish* an agreement with parents, children, and caregivers concerning open communication. At the onset it is important to acknowledge one's own discomfort with the feelings about death and the dying child. These powerful feelings could sabotage communication.

2. *Engage* the child at the opportune time. Often an unexpected procedure could be the impetus behind the death discussion. Being mindful of overt behavioral reactions may lead to an opportunity to discuss feelings the child is struggling with.

3. *Explore* the child's present understanding of their illness and invite questions. This allows for any misconceptions and misunderstandings to be corrected and validates the child's natural curiosity.

4. *Explain* medical information regarding the child's treatment protocol. Naturally, conveying this information is predicated on the developmental level of the child. Open-ended questions are a useful tool in allowing the child to control their knowledge intake. "What would you like to know?" "What is your biggest worry?" "What would make you happy right now?" are a few questions that address the medical and psychosocial concerns of the child.

5. *Empathize* with the child's emotional reactions. Creating a safe environment in which the child can express feelings of both anger and angst is critical for the child's well-being. Validating a child's reactions with empathy and clarification instead of minimizing them with platitudes can foster the relationship.

6. *Encourage* the child by reassuring him or her that you will be there to listen and be a continued support. Feeling alone and isolated are sources of anxiety for the dying child. Acknowledging to the child that cure is not possible and their life is limited provides the child with a new hope system that their final days will be pain-free, comfortable, and they will not be alone.

It should be noted that established family communication patterns and religious and cultural beliefs profoundly influence the style in which parents can exercise these guidelines with their dying child. However, when a child is provided with an opportunity to communicate, it allows for healing and control of fears.

The clinical needs of the adolescent with cancer are not significantly different from those of the child with cancer. Adaptation to treatment and secondary losses are particularly challenging for the adolescent. Depending on the age of the adolescent, they must cope with changes in peer relationships; self-image; prolonged absences from school or college; leave from a job; reestablishing oneself in the nuclear family; and ambivalence about the future.

Unique to the adolescent psychosocial needs is the fact that teens are living in a world governed by technology. Adolescents form one of the most active groups of Internet users. Cell phones, BlackBerries, laptops, and social networking sites are a few of the mainstream tools teenagers use daily for communication. Adolescents skillfully navigate through the Internet, exploring information on healthcare issues concerning exercise, sexual health, and alcohol and drugs. Developmentally, adolescents are known to have difficulty forming relationships with professional healthcare workers (Klein, Wilson, McNulty, Kapphahn, & Collins, 1999). Beresford and Sloper (2003) concluded that while adolescents may seek out medical information from health professionals, they seek out friends and other adolescents with similar diagnoses for their psychosocial concerns and questions.

Katie, a 15-year-old home hospice patient, was recently hospitalized with severe abdominal pain. Although her procedure to relieve the pain was not scheduled immediately, Katie found comfort in using her laptop to instant message (IM) with friends at home. This tool allowed her to process her fears with the people she trusts the most—her friends. When I asked her why she didn't use her cell phone, she responded, "I don't have any privacy to talk on the phone with my friends." Family and hospital staff were constantly in and out of Katie's hospital room, providing little alone time for Katie to connect with friends.

Numerous research studies have been and continue to be conducted on the use of Internet resources with adolescents. In one study (Skinner, Biscope, Poland, & Goldberg, 2003), the participants regarded the Internet as a combined communication, entertainment, and information medium. Health advice and treatment protocols were explored at any time of the day or evening. Adolescents can travel beyond their own life experience using the Internet and access pertinent information regarding health and well-being (Gray, Klein, Noyce, Sesselberg, & Cantrill, 2005). The adolescent quest for knowledge on the Internet, however, can sometimes be of limited usefulness. Many adolescents felt frustrated when their search skills failed them and they were unable to access more information. However, as adolescents become more informed about their disease and assume an active role in their treatments, the Internet positions them to make educated and informed choices together with their parents and medical staff.

Remaining anonymous while searching the Web is an attractive component to the adolescent. Adolescents are attracted to cancer support chat rooms because they aren't immediately required to disclose personal information. As the Internet relationship develops and trust is established with other adolescents with cancer, he or she is prepared to share more personal information about him or herself. Validating their cancer journey by sharing stories, crises, hopes, and dreams with another adolescent can be a healing process.

Not that dissimilar from adolescents, many parents utilize the Internet for treatment information. One parent told me that it has empowered her to advocate for her daughter when medical staff is remiss in explaining certain medical procedures. Another parent researched children's palliative care and hospice online and made an educated decision to ask for services after reviewing the literature. John S. Rolland believes, "Continual adaptation and role change is implicit. Increasing strain on family caretakers is caused by both the risks of exhaustion and the continual addition of new caretaking tasks over time. Family flexibility both in terms of internal role reorganization and their willingness to use outside resources are at a premium" (Rolland, 1988).

As the child and adolescent transition from curative treatments to palliative and hospice care, their psychosocial needs begin to change. Nicholas, 5 years old and dying at home with hospice, spent his last days in his own bed surrounded by his immediate family: mother, father, younger sister, and grandparents. Individual family members alternately stroked Nicholas's head and held his hands. In a particularly religious family, Nicholas announced shortly before his death that he was "scared to meet God." When questioned by his grandmother, he said he was afraid he wouldn't have his favorite pajamas on. This tender and teachable moment allowed his parents to reassure Nicholas that he would be wearing his Spider Man pajamas when he meets God.

Three days before 7-year-old Eliza died, she spent most every second wrapped safely in her father's arms in bed. Whenever an opportunity presented itself, such as when Eliza was sleeping, her father would gingerly climb out of bed. It was not long before he was summoned by Eliza or a family member to return. On the day of her death, the hospice nurse shared with me that Eliza instructed her father that she needed to show her mother, who had died 3 years earlier, her missing tooth. Eliza's father courageously gave her permission to "go play with Mommy in heaven." Eliza died seconds later.

The night before lapsing into her coma, 19-year-old Tina had the strength to crawl into bed with her younger sister. The physical closeness, snuggled up with her sister, was a confirmation that she was still present and alive. The following morning, Tina, like Eliza, needed a parent to give her permission. It is important not to disregard the request for permission to die. Tina's most notable wish to her mother was, "You have to help other people. Other people can't go through this." Since Tina's death 4 years ago, a foundation has been established in her name to address the psychosocial needs of the young adult with ovarian cancer.

As 15-year-old Katie has become aware that death is imminent, she has begun to actively journal and scrapbook. This medium allows her a safe modality to continue to connect with friends and family and leave a powerful legacy behind. On home visits, Katie is often relaxing on the couch with a friend or her younger sister. As she engages in art experientials, her sister and mother are present by her side, fully mindful of their time together.

Parents hear all types of responses when the medical staff has exhausted all curative treatment options. "It is the best we can do." "We can't do anymore." "Have you thought about hospice?" These are just a few of the responses parents have relayed to me. The defining moment when a parent decides to utilize palliative care and hospice is very different for each family. Palliative care and hospice enhances the quality of the end of life. The American Academy of Pediatrics defines palliative care as including the control of pain and other symptoms and addresses the psychological, social, or spiritual problems of children living with life-threatening or terminal conditions (Committee on Bioethics and Committee on Hospital Care, 2000).

The palliative care model is also defined as a practice born to address the unmet needs of children suffering from serious disease. Pediatric palliative care focuses on the essentials of life itself: the basic needs to have meaningful relationships and a sense of completion in one's life—a sense of meaning. These are basic needs of the human psyche and apply to children as well as adults (Cassell, 1982). Palliative and hospice support is a humanistic model that reflects the needs of the individual and family. Guided by a strong sense of hope, many parents continue to grapple with the transition to palliative and hospice care for their dying child.

Parents' resiliency and the ability to exhibit unyielding strength in the face of adversity can be supported by the palliative care and hospice staff.

Marianne Walsh, MS, CT, received her master of science degree in art therapy and completed the post-graduate program in thanatology from the College of New Rochelle. She is coordinator of hospice care in Westchester & Putnam's Caring Circle Bereavement Program. As a practicing art therapist with hospice care, she works directly with the patients and their families at the end of life as well as bereavement. Ms. Walsh is an active member of the Northern Westchester & Putnam BOCES Regional Crisis Team and has presented at the New York Association of School Psychologists Conferences. Over the last 8 years, she has been involved with the Westchester Community Networks Program, providing bereavement outreach and support to children and adolescents in the school environment and their homes.

REFERENCES

Beale, E. A., Baile, W. F., & Aaron, J. (2005). Silence is not golden: Communicating with children dying of cancer. *Journal of Clinical Oncology, 23*, 3629–3631.

Beresford, B., & Sloper, P. (2003). Chronically ill adolescents' experiences of communicating with doctors: A qualitative study. *Journal of Adolescent Health, 33*(3), 172–179.

Bertoia, J. (1993). *Drawings from a dying child: Insights from a Jungian perspective.* New York: Routledge.

Cassell, E. J. (1982). The nature of suffering and the goals of medicine. *New England Journal of Medicine, 302,* 639–645.

Committee on Bioethics and Committee on Hospital Care: American Academy of Pediatrics. (2000). Palliative care for children. *Pediatrics, 106,* 351–357.

Councill, T. (1993). Art therapy with pediatric cancer patients: Helping normal children cope with abnormal circumstances. *Art Therapy, 10*(2), 78–87.

Doka, K. J. (1995). Talking to children about illness. In K. J. Doka (Ed.), *Children mourning, mourning children.* Washington, DC: Hospice Foundation of America.

Faulkner, K. W. (1993). Children's understanding of death. In A. Armstrong-Dailey & S. Zarbock-Goltzer (Eds.), *Hospice care for children.* New York: Oxford University Press.

Faulkner, K. W. (1997). Talking about death with a dying child. *American Journal of Nursing, 97,* 64–69.

Gray, N. J., Klein, J. D., Noyce, P. R., Sesselberg, T. S., & Cantrill, J. A. (2005). Health information-seeking behaviour in adolescence: The place of the Internet. *Social Science and Medicine, 60,* 1467–1478.

Hadlock, D. C. (1985). The hospice: Intensive care of a different kind. *Seminars in Oncology, 12,* 357–367.

Hinds, P. S., Oakes, L., Furman, W., Foppiano, P., Olson, M. S., Quargnenti, A., et al. (1997). Decision making by parents and healthcare professionals when considering continued care for pediatric patients with cancer. *Oncology Nursing Forum, 24*(9), 1523–1528.

Klein, J. D., Wilson, K. M., McNulty, M., Kapphahn, C., & Collins, K. S. (1999). Access to medical care for adolescents: Results from the commonwealth Fund Survey of the Health of Adolescent Girls. *Journal of Adolescent Health, 25,* 120–130.

Levy, M. H. (1985). The palliative-curative interface. *Seminars in Oncology, 12,* 355–356.

Ries, L. A. G., Eisner, M. P., Kosary, C. L., Hankey, B. F., Miller, B. A., Clegg, L., et al. (2004). *SEER cancer statistics review, 1975–2001.* Bethesda, MD: National Cancer Institute.

Rolland, J. S. (1988). *Chronic disorders of the family.* New York: Routledge.

Rubin, J. A. (1984). *The art of art therapy.* New York: Routledge.

Skinner, H. A., Biscope, S., Poland, B., & Goldberg, E. (2003). How adolescents use technology for health information: Implications for practitioners. *Journal of Medical Internet Research, 5*(4), e32.

Sourkes, B. M. (1992). The child with a life-threatening illness. In J. Brandell (Ed.), *Countertransference in psychotherapy with children and adolescents,* pp. 267–284. New York: Jason Aronson.

Whittam, E. H. (1993). Terminal care of the dying child. *Cancer, 71,* 3450–3462.

Personal Perspective: Vivienne's Story

Mary Martin

What started as a routine checkup in June 2008 for my 2-month-old daughter, Vivienne Esmé, turned into a parent's worst nightmare. Within a day, Vivienne was scheduled for brain shunt surgery. Within the next few weeks, she was diagnosed with an atypical teratoid rhabdoid tumor, an extremely rare form of cancer affecting her brain, spine, and one kidney. From the beginning, my husband and I were told that curative treatment had no chance of success. Instead of worrying about a fever from standard immunizations, we spent the next month coming to grips with terms like *palliative care* and learning how to properly dose morphine using an oral syringe.

Floored, we left home and spent time with family in Maine, where Vivi learned to laugh. During this time, we consulted with various neuro-oncology groups, including Children's Hospital of Philadelphia, Memorial Sloan Kettering, New York University, and St. Jude Children's Research Hospital. After lengthy and heartfelt discussions together and with a grief counselor, we realized that giving up was not an option. In a whirlwind, we packed our things and moved to Memphis for brain surgery, kidney surgery, and chemotherapy.

The concept of withholding curative treatment from our daughter and, as we then viewed it, simply allowing her to die was unfathomable to us. On the other hand, we also strongly reacted to comments that putting a very small baby through chemotherapy might be, as one oncologist said, akin to torture. From the beginning, we committed ourselves to maintaining the right balance between pursuing a cure and preserving Vivienne's quality of life. That meant that even as we attempted curative treatment, Vivi's comfort and happiness would always be our first priority. We began aggressive experimental treatment, watching Vivienne's side effects, her pain level, and her ability to engage with and enjoy the world around her. We walked a delicate line between maintaining hope for the future and accepting the reality of her prognosis.

After the surgery in August removed the vast majority of the brain tumor, Vivienne became more alert, comfortable, and engaged. When the initial courses of chemotherapy produced a similar reaction, we were thrilled to have pursued treatment with a curative intent and palliative effect. At all times, our realistic treatment goal was to extend Vivi's life for as long as we could. We fought hard to destroy the tumor but never forgot that we had to allow Vivi to live for today. Having maintained that goal, we have memories of Vivienne's fascination with panda bears at the Memphis Zoo and pictures of her enjoying the sights and sounds of the Children's Museum of Memphis. Our family blog documents Vivi kicking her feet fast when excited, opening her Christmas presents, watching fish in the aquarium, and many other baby adventures. We look back on our decisions with peace and acceptance, knowing that we did the best we could to give our daughter a life filled with as much fun as we could create.

After 6 months of treatment, Vivienne's cancer became resistant to chemotherapy. In January 2009, she suffered a seizure and a follow-up MRI showed many new tumors developing. This was the second time the world dropped out from underneath us. While we had always attempted to remain realistic in our hopes, being told a second time to withhold curative treatment was a crushing blow.

In the week after receiving this news, we worked with Vivienne's doctors to understand whether there were any surgical or other reasonable treatment protocols that might buy Vivi more time to grow, play, and be loved. This was an amplification of the first weeks after her diagnosis, when we chased rainbows searching online for a Hail Mary pass. Some people pointed us toward different "alternative" treatments. Others queried why we couldn't pursue radiation. (Vivienne was too young.) A few well-meaning souls forwarded stories of holy miracles, untested theories, Vitamin C, and other long shots. We were haunted with fear that we would decide against pursuing some unusual treatment that years later might be proven as a definitive cure.

On the other hand, we refused to inflict truly hopeless treatment on a sweet, happy baby just to make ourselves feel better for doing something. Our promises made months earlier in the neonatal intensive care unit in Philadelphia bound us never to act in a way that would help our emotions, but hurt our daughter. Putting her needs first, we concluded that the scenario in January was different than that of the previous July. Vivienne's tiny body had battled through two brain surgeries, a kidney removal, and 6 months of aggressive chemotherapy. She was a happy, outgoing, active baby, but the side effects were beginning to show. The chemotherapy had caused a full loss of hearing in one ear, recurring infections, the need for a barrage of supportive medication, and other effects. We decided against becoming more aggressive when Vivienne's body was already hurting and instead decided to help relieve that pain for her and allow her to live with joy.

The difference in our knowledge and acceptance of Vivienne's cancer was a key point in deciding that hospice-only care was a positive step in January 2009 after deciding against it in July 2008. Having experienced chemotherapy and its impact on Vivi and knowing that we had fought hard for her to have a longer life, we were able to see when enough was enough. What seemed like medical nay-saying in July appeared measured, reasonable, and responsible in January. Knowing the suffering that treatment could bring, with the resistance to chemotherapy making further success even less likely, we viewed the decision to move to hospice care as fighting for Vivi's comfort rather than giving up the fight for her life.

With that in mind, we brought Vivi home on a donated flight in a private jet and began meeting with our hospice professionals. This was as positive as circumstances would allow, because the caregivers we spoke with carefully listened to our needs and educated us in an appropriate way. We wanted to avoid suffering for Vivi but allow her to have experiences and enjoy life as long as possible. After stating these goals, we learned appropriate pain level evaluation techniques. Nurse visits were scheduled as infrequently or as often as we wished, which allowed us both privacy and the comfort of assistance with decision making and medical needs. This approach allowed us to plan family events and fun activities for Vivi, including a homecoming queen party and plenty of play time. Our hospice nurses, who were saints to us, accepted hysterical, scared calls at very odd hours and stood by with advice to help us manage every problem.

When Vivienne passed away very early in the morning on February 17, 2009, I was numb and in shock, knowing that the moments of that day would be branded into my mind for life. But thanks to making positive decisions throughout Vivienne's life and carefully balancing the transition from curative to palliative care, my husband and I look back without self-recrimination on the positive moments that the team of caregivers (family and professionals alike) worked together to provide for Vivi. Finding personal and family peace in the tragedy of a child's terminal illness is a very individual path, and we appreciate the doctors and professionals who supported and guided us to make the decisions that worked for our family's needs and personal values.

Mary Martin *lives in Bucks County, Pennsylvania, with her husband Justin. Mary, a structured settlement lawyer, and Justin, a floral designer, gave birth to their only child, Vivienne, on April 24, 2008. After Vivienne was diagnosed with brain cancer, the Martin family moved to Memphis, Tennessee, for care at St. Jude Children's Research Hospital. Both Mary and Justin have found peace in giving Vivienne's life meaning by sharing her story in hopes of helping other families, primarily through their family blogs "Viva la Vivi" and "A Big Sister in Heaven." Although Mary and Justin are now infertile after injuries during Vivi's birth, they are planning to bring more children into their family in the future.*

CHAPTER 12

Facing Cancer: The Gender Dimension

Neil Thompson

T he literature relating to cancer is of understandably significant proportions, covering a wide range of biological, psychological, social, and spiritual issues. One aspect that has received relatively little attention is that of gender—the ways in which men and women may experience cancer differently because of the complex array of factors that construct gender roles, expectations, and reactions. This chapter is therefore one small contribution to putting the gender dimension of cancer on the agenda.

The chapter is divided into three parts: a short discussion of the significance of cancer; a consideration of gender as a factor in people's general lives and, more specifically, in relation to encounters with cancer; and how the intersection of cancer and gender has implications for identity, for our sense of who we are and how we fit into the wider world.

THE SIGNIFICANCE OF CANCER

The very mention of the word "cancer" is something that can strike fear into people's hearts. Hoffman (2004) captures this point well:

> Walking into the cancer clinic for the first time was simply terrifying. Symbolically and literally, we crossed from the healthy and secure world, as we had known it, into a world of suffering, uncertainty and fear. (p. 58)

This significance is also quite broad in its impact, affecting not only patients and their families and friends, but also professional staff involved in providing treatment and care. How people respond to the pressures involved will vary enormously, sometimes serving to ease the pressures, sometimes making them worse. An instance of the latter would be a professional who, in attempting to keep his or her own feelings under control, comes across as cold and uncaring to others. Hoffman gives an example of this in describing a doctor in the following terms: "He bound his own anxiety by bombarding families with far more scientific data than we needed, wanted, or could handle" (p. 59).

THE SIGNIFICANCE OF GENDER

While cancer is clearly a very significant phenomenon, so too is gender. As we shall see below, when we combine the two, the significance is even greater. I shall begin by discussing the role of gender in general before commenting specifically on how it relates to cancer.

General

While sex is a matter of biology, gender is a psychosocial phenomenon. That is, it is a combination of psychological and sociological factors. Gender can be understood as part of what women and men *do* to express their identity. Gender shapes how we speak (Sunderland, 2004); how we feel (Parkinson, Fischer, & Manstead, 2005); how we behave (Connell, 2002); and therefore, how we care. In terms of caring, there is, of course, a balance to be struck between clinical detachment and emotional honesty. There is now a growing literature on the relationships between gender and emotion (Fischer, 2000). In a similar vein, the work of Martin and Doka (2000) has shown that gender is also a significant factor in relation to how loss and grief are experienced and dealt with. This, of course, is very significant when it comes to considering the relationship between gender and cancer.

Specific to Cancer

There are clear biological sex differences in respect to cancer. Consider, for example, the existence of cervical cancer in women and prostate cancer in men (Rice, 2005). But there are also socially constructed gender differences. One particularly significant example is the occurrence of breast cancer in men. Breast cancer is generally assumed to be a female phenomenon. According to the Dana-Farber Cancer Institute (www.dana-farber.org), male breast cancer accounts for less than 1% of breast carcinomas (although it needs to be recognized that this is still significant, with 2,030 new cases in the United States in 2007 and 450 deaths). Having to cope with cancer is, of course, difficult enough for everyone affected, but for men with breast cancer there is the additional challenge of feeling alienated in a context that conflicts with what their gender socialization has taught them. The case in Practice Focus 1 on page 153 illustrates this very well.

At the other end of the spectrum is prostate cancer, a form of cancer that applies to men only. Prostate cancer is the most commonly diagnosed cancer

Simon, age 34, is living with breast cancer. He has been treated with chemotherapy and radiotherapy and is now on hormone therapy. He describes how isolated and confused he felt when he was diagnosed. He remembers the breast care clinic being a very female environment with pink ribbons and support groups targeting women; he felt very uncomfortable sitting with other women in the clinic. Simon felt embarrassed about having breast cancer and was unable to share with his friends and colleagues the true nature of his illness. He described the side effects of his treatment as shameful, as they had affected his energy levels and sex life.

Simon's partner, Jill, found his reaction to his illness frustrating, as he would not talk to her about how he was feeling. She was concerned that he was having angry outbursts and taking risks, such as driving fast and drinking increasing amounts of alcohol. Jill tried to encourage Simon to talk about how the death of his mother to breast cancer when he was 11 years old may be affecting him. Also she thought that he was worrying that he may have passed on his hereditary illness to their young son. However, Simon did not want to talk; to him, what was the point?

Simon and Jill came to the agreement that they could help each other cope by agreeing to a plan of action to deal with living with cancer. They decided that their focus should be how to support each other in staying well and getting physically fit again. Simon found motivation and purpose through a Web site-based male breast cancer support group that organized sports events to raise money for breast cancer research. This helped him to come to terms with his illness in ways that did not compromise his sense of masculinity.

in the United Kingdom. Some 35,000 men are diagnosed each year and 1 man dies from prostate cancer each hour (Prostate Cancer Charity, 2009). Despite the absence of the conflict between masculine gender expectations and the predominantly feminine world of breast cancer treatment, men with prostate cancer still face significant gender challenges. For example, a very common treatment is hormone therapy. In 8 out of 10 cases, men under this treatment experience erectile dysfunction and 50% of them report serious issues related to mental well-being (such as depression, loss of confidence, and cognitive problems) (ibid.). The case of Joe in Practice Focus 2 on page 155 illustrates well the difficulties.

The two practice focus examples are rich illustrations of how gender can be understood to construct the experience of illness (Dale and Altschuler, 2002). Similarly, in a study of the experiences of the middle-aged children of people who have died from cancer, the researchers concluded that gender accounted for most of the differences in those experiences (Moss, Resch, & Moss, 1997).

To pursue further the theme of men and masculinity, it is important to consider what society expects of men. For example, Lattanzi-Licht (1999) points out that men are generally expected to be task oriented. This echoes Martin and Doka's (2000) work on gendered patterns of grieving and the recognition of a preference among most men for an instrumental style of grieving.

Masculinity can also be a key factor in terms of a reluctance to seek help. For example, Smith, Pope, and Botha (2005) indicate that men's reluctance to seek medical help can potentially be disastrous because of the reduced effectiveness of delayed treatment. In addition, a research report by the National Cancer Intelligence Network (2009) makes reference to the fact that men are less likely to have a healthy lifestyle, thus adding to their susceptibility to the disease (and other complicating factors).

However, the relationship between cancer and gender is not something that simply relates to men. For example, recent research by the Target Ovarian Cancer organization indicates that many women are dying unnecessarily from ovarian cancer because physicians sometimes miss the symptoms (Target Ovarian Cancer, 2009). The point I am trying to emphasize is not that there are specifically masculine dimensions to cancer. Rather, I am making the broader point that gender is a significant issue in relation to cancer for both men and women.

It is also important to recognize that some cancer-related issues affect both men and women, albeit in different ways. For example, Patenaude (2000)

Joe, age 66, was diagnosed with prostate cancer with bone secondaries; his treatment involved hormone therapy. Joe was referred for psychotherapy by his specialist nurse, as he appeared to be depressed and not coping with his illness. Joe and his wife, Myra, explained to the therapist that his personality had completely changed since the illness. He had no drive to do anything. His relationships with Myra and children had become strained and he thought he was suffering from some sort of brain disorder because his cognitive functioning in doing ordinary daily tasks had declined.

Joe's physician had prescribed antidepressants, but he had not taken them because he did not think of himself as depressed. He still wanted to engage in his life, but had lost the ability to do so. He felt distressed because he did not feel like the man he used to be. He had always taken charge of the household finances and made the major decisions in family life. He had poor libido and was suffering from erectile dysfunction. Myra tearfully talked about how she felt robbed of the intimate part of her life and she could not understand why Joe had withdrawn so completely from her. She was fearful of making decisions she had never made before, and Joe was not able to guide her.

Joe was able to tell Myra that his sense of masculinity and what being a husband meant to him had been totally challenged. He felt useless and guilty. He withdrew because he did not know how else to cope. The therapist was able to talk with Joe and Myra about the impact of hormone therapy. This, together with the feelings of loss that come with the diagnosis of a life-limiting illness were, of course, contributing to this painful situation.

Joe and Myra agreed that they would talk with their oncologist about other treatment options that, although they might shorten his life, would enable him to function in his role and restore what they felt to be important in their relationship.

makes an interesting comment on how reactions to the cancer of one's parents have a significant gender dimension:

> Not surprisingly, research has shown that the emotional distress is greatest on a child when the parent of the same sex is ill. Compas et al. (1994) found that adolescent girls, the most distressed of all groups of children and young adults whose parent is ill, were most distressed when their mother was ill. Adolescent boys were also most distressed when their father was the cancer patient. Wellisch et al. (1992) also found that women who had been adolescents at the time their mother was being diagnosed with breast cancer were more distressed than women who had been younger at the time their parent became ill. More research is needed on the cause of this association, but we can speculate that a contributing factor is the threat to the growing identification of the adolescent. Witnessing the physical and emotional vulnerability of the same-sex parent may make them more hesitant to accept the changes in their own maturing bodies. (p. 246)

Once again, then, we see that gender is a key factor relating to cancer. But there are also wider gender issues in relation to organizational and other such contextual factors. For example, consider the role of hospice in cancer care. The hospice movement was founded on the idea of openness to death and mortality (Seale, 1989), but men and women may react differently to the expectation to be open to what are, after all, very emotionally charged matters.

Recognizing that loss and grief occur in response to any major loss and not just to death (Thompson, 2002), it is important to note that the initial grief relating to cancer is likely to occur perhaps long before the grief associated with the death. Returning once more to the work of Martin and Doka (2000) around gender-differentiated approaches to loss, we can surmise that responses to the onset and diagnosis of cancer are therefore also likely to follow gender patterns. To fail to recognize the grief associated with encountering a diagnosis of cancer and to fail to acknowledge and address the gender dimensions of that grief is likely to have the effect of rendering such grief doubly disenfranchised (Doka, 1989).

The grief associated with cancer will, of course, need to be dealt with. Scholars and professionals in the field of loss and grief are increasingly recognizing the central role of "meaning reconstruction" (Neimeyer, 2001).

This involves the development of a new "narrative"—a story or framework of meaning that helps the grieving individual make sense of the profoundly unsettling transition he or she is going through. It needs to be recognized that such meaning reconstruction will be channeled through gender expectations. The new narrative that develops cannot be independent of the influence of gender because, as we noted earlier in this chapter, gender shapes how we think, feel, and behave.

Pitceathly and Maguire (2000) have also noted further gender difference in relation to cancer, adding more weight to the argument that gender is a very significant factor to take into consideration when responding to the challenges of cancer. They argue that

> Gender differences have been noticed in the influence one partner has on the other's adjustment. Northouse et al. (1995) and Hannum et al. (1991) suggested that breast cancer patients were more influenced by their husbands' adjustment than husbands were influenced by wives, but in Keller et al.'s study (1996) with a mixed cancer population, male partners' distress was moderated by other factors. (p. 139)

There should be no doubt, then, that gender and cancer intertwine in various important ways. One aspect of this that we have not yet considered is that of identity.

THE IMPLICATIONS FOR IDENTITY

It has long been recognized that identity is gendered. That is, who we are depends very much on the influence of gender expectations (Lawler, 2008). Cancer is also significant in terms of identity. As Stacey (1997) so tellingly comments: "Cancer is the *self* at war with *self*. Thus, surely one's identity is at stake (on trial?) with the onset of such a disease" (pp. 62–63).

Rhodes, Iedema, and Scheeres (2007) argue that identity is "embodied." That is, identity cannot be entirely separated from bodily experience. When cancer arises, the individual faces a "transition to body-object" (Lawton, 2000). The focus of attention switches from the person as a whole to the body of the person. Given the way cancer ravages the human body and the fact that much of the treatment to defeat cancer can also have detrimental effects on the body, there will clearly be identity implications arising from cancer. (The two case illustrations earlier in this chapter also echo this idea.)

Little, Paul, Jordens, and Sayers (2002) emphasize the impact of cancer on identity:

> We believe that the experience of surviving cancer illness can be better understood by examining the discourses of personal identity that appear in narratives of cancer experienced and survived, and of cancer illness observed and cared for. We believe, furthermore, that surviving cancer produces changes in the sense of personal identity, and it is important to understand these changes if one is to understand what it is to be a cancer survivor. (pp. 170–172)

So, at a time a person's identity faces changes as a result of cancer, what role can gender be seen to play? What are the implications of this for maintaining a gendered identity, of continuing to *do* gender in ways that are expected of us? These are important questions that merit much fuller treatment than I am able to give here. However, it is worth noting that at least one study of cancer-related experiences found little of note in relation to gender. The comments of Lawton (2000) on this matter are instructive:

> It appears that one of the principal reasons why gendered differences were not prominent in this study is because patients often experienced a disinvestment of their masculinity or femininity even in the early stages of their illness and deterioration. (p. 166)

The irony here, then, is that gender differences appear not to have featured because gender identity was somehow submerged by the changes occurring as a result of cancer. This in itself makes a major point about the significance of identity when cancer enters the scene: A key part of who we are (our gender identity) no longer seems to feature. This can be seen as part of a broader process of depersonalization or dehumanization that so often occurs when a person becomes seriously ill.

The focus in this chapter has been on gender. However, one final point to note is that, because gender differences are socially constructed, they also need to be seen in the context of other social structural factors. Gender does not operate independently of such factors as class, race/ethnicity, sexuality, age, or disability, but rather interacts closely with them in complex ways (Thompson, 2003). Interested readers may consult Candib (2002) and Tamasese and Waldegrave (1996) as good starting points.

CONCLUSION

This chapter has explored the relationship between cancer and gender. Its basic argument has been that, in order to gain a comprehensive understanding of cancer and its treatment, we need to take account of gender. "Explored" is a key word, insofar as what can realistically be covered in one short chapter cannot be described as comprehensive or exhaustive. Clearly, there is much more to be said and written about this important, but relatively neglected aspect of health care.

To conclude, I offer brief comments for three different sets of stakeholders to draw out the lessons to be learned from what I have tried to express in this chapter.

Scholars: What emerges clearly from a consideration of the relationship between cancer and gender is that there is considerable scope for research and theory development in this area. It is to be hoped that this brief overview will play a part in stimulating such much-needed development.

Caring professionals: Working in the field of cancer care is in itself a demanding undertaking. However, we need to make sure that the efforts that go into such important and valuable work are not misdirected or even counterproductive because they failed to pay adequate attention to gender differences in particular and the significance of gender in people's lives in general. Hoffman (2004) argues that: "More than anything else, patients and families need to know that people care. In the end, that is what matters" (p. 71). To ensure that caring efforts achieve optimal outcomes, we therefore need to make sure that we are listening to what a more sophisticated understanding of gender is saying about people's lives.

Patients, families, and other caregivers: Encountering cancer can be confusing, disorientating, and, of course, unsettling. The better the understanding of what is happening, the stronger a position the individual will be in when it comes to dealing with the pressures and challenges involved. An awareness and fuller grasp of the role of gender can be seen to be part of the understanding that is needed.

ACKNOWLEDGMENTS

I am very grateful for the support and assistance I have received in the preparation of this chapter from my friends Mary Tehan, Irene Renzenbrink, and especially Denise Bevan.

Neil Thompson, PhD, is director of Avenue Consulting Ltd. (www. avenueconsulting.co.uk), a company based in Wales offering training and consultancy services in relation to well-being—especially workplace well-being and more broadly, social well-being. He has held full or honorary professorships at four U.K. universities and has been a speaker at conferences and seminars in Europe, Hong Kong, India, Australia, Canada, and the United States. He has over 100 publications to his name, including several best-selling textbooks. His latest book is Loss, Grief and Trauma in the Workplace (Baywood, 2009). He is the editor of Illness, Crisis & Loss and is the editor-in-chief of the online community Well-being Zone (www.well-beingzone.com) and is a member of the International Work Group on Death, Dying, and Bereavement. His personal Web site is www.neilthompson.info. He is a sought-after conference speaker, consultant, and workshop facilitator.

REFERENCES

Candib, L. M. (2002). Truth telling and advance planning at the end of life: Problems with autonomy in a multicultural world. *Families, Systems & Health, 20*(3), pp. 213–228.

Compas, B. E., Worsham, N. L., Epping-Jordan, J. E., Grant, K. E., Mireault, G., Howell, D. C., et al. (1994). When mom or dad has cancer: Markers of psychological distress in cancer patients, spouses and children. *Health Psychology, 13*, 507–515.

Connell, R. W. (2002). *Gender.* Cambridge, UK: Polity Press.

Dale, B., & Altschuler, J. (2002). Different language/different gender: Narratives of inclusion and exclusion. In R. K. Papadopoulos & J. Byng-Hall (Eds.), *Multiple voices: Narrative in systemic family psychotherapy* (2nd ed.). London: Karnac.

Doka, K. (Ed.). (1989). *Disenfranchised grief.* New York: Jossey Bass.

Fischer, A. H. (Ed.). (2000). *Gender and emotion: Social psychological perspectives.* Cambridge, UK: Cambridge University Press.

Hannum, J. W., Giese-Davis, J., Harding, K. & Hatfield, A. K. (1991). Effects of individual and marital variables on coping with cancer. *Journal of Psychosocial Oncology, 9*, 1–20.

Hoffman, R. (2004). The loss of a child to cancer: From case to caseworker. In J. Berzoff & P. Silverman (Eds.), *Living with dying: A handbook for end-of-life healthcare practitioners.* New York: Columbia University Press.

Keller, M., Henrich, G., Sellschopp, A., & Beutel, M. (1996). Between stress and support: Spouses of cancer patients. In L. Baider, C. L. Cooper, & A. Kaplan De-Nour (Eds.), *Cancer and the family* (2nd ed.). Chichester and New York: Wiley.

Lattanzi-Licht, M. E. (1999). Grief in the workplace: Supporting the grieving employee. In J. D. Davidson & K. J. Doka (Eds.), *Living with grief: At work, at school, at worship*. Washington, DC: Hospice Foundation of America.

Lawler, S. (2008). *Identity: Sociological perspectives*. Cambridge, UK: Polity Press.

Lawton, J. (2000). *The dying process: Patients' experiences of palliative care*. New York: Routledge.

Little, M., Paul, K., Jordens, C. F. C. & Sayers, E. J. (2002). Survivorship and discourses of identity. *Psycho-Oncology, 11*, 170–178.

Martin, T. L., & Doka, K. J. (2000). *Men don't cry... women do: Transcending gender stereotypes of grief*. Philadelphia: Brunner/Mazel.

Moss, M. S., Resch, N., & Moss, S. Z. (1997). The role of gender in middle-age children's responses to parent death. *Omega: Journal of Death and Dying, 35*, 43–65.

National Cancer Intelligence Network. (2009). *The Excess Burden of Cancer in Men in the UK*. Retrieved July 1, 2009 from http://publications. cancerresearchuk.org/WebRoot/crukstoredb/CRUK_PDFs/CSNCINMALE.pdf

Neimeyer, R. A. (Ed.). (2001). *Meaning reconstruction and the experience of loss*. Washington, DC: American Psychological Association.

Northouse, L., Dorris, G. & Charron-Moore, C. (1995). Factors affecting couples' adjustment to recurrent breast cancer. *Social Science and Medicine, 41*, 69–76.

Parkinson, B., Fischer, A. H., & Manstead, A. S. R. (2005). *Emotion in social relations*. New York: Psychology Press.

Patenaude, A. F. (2000). A different normal: Reactions of children and adolescents to the diagnosis of cancer in a parent. In L. Baider, C. L. Cooper, & A. K. De-Nour (Eds.), *Cancer and the family* (2nd ed.). Chichester and New York: Wiley.

Pitceathly, C., & Maguire, P. (2000). Preventing affective disorders in partners of cancer patients: An intervention study. In L. Baider, C. L. Cooper, & A. K. De-Nour (Eds.), *Cancer and the family* (2nd ed.). Chichester and New York: Wiley.

Prostate Cancer Charity. (2009). *Hampered by hormones? Addressing the needs of men with prostate cancer*. London: The Prostate Cancer Charity.

Rhodes, C., Iedema, R., & Scheeres, H. (2007). Identity, surveillance and resistance. In A. Pullen, N. Beech, & D. Sims (Eds.), *Exploring identity: Concepts and methods*. Basingstoke and New York: Palgrave Macmillan.

Rice, K. (2005). *Gender impact assessment: Cancer*. Melbourne: Women's Health Victoria.

Seale, C. (1989). What happens in hospices: A review of research evidence. *Social Science and Medicine, 28*(6), 551–559.

Smith, L. K., Pope, C. & Botha, J. L. (2005). Patients' help-seeking experiences and delay in presentation: A qualitative synthesis. *Lancet, 366*, 825–831.

Stacey, J. (1997). *Teratologies: A cultural study of cancer*. London: Routledge.

Sunderland, J. (2004). *Gendered discourses*. Basingstoke and New York: Palgrave Macmillan.

Tamasese, K., & Waldegrave, C. (1996). Cultural and gender accountability in the "Just Therapy" approach. In C. McLean, M. Carey, & C. White (Eds.), *Men's ways of being*. London: Westview Press.

Target Ovarian Cancer. (2009). *The Target Ovarian Cancer pathfinder study: Preliminary results*. Retrieved July 1, 2009 from http://www.targetovarian.org.uk

Thompson, N. (Ed.). (2002). *Loss and grief: A guide for human services professionals*. Basingstoke and New York: Palgrave Macmillan.

Thompson, N. (2003). *Promoting equality* (2nd ed.). Basingstoke and New York: Palgrave Macmillan.

Wellisch, D. K., Gritz, E. R., Schain, W., Wang, H. J., & Siau, J. (1992). Psychological functioning of daughters of breast cancer patients part II: Characterizing the distressed daughter of the cancer patient. *Psychosomatics, 33*, 171–179.

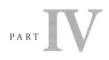

Grief and Cancer

A central principle of hospice is that the family or intimate network is the unit of care. This recognizes that life-threatening illnesses such as cancer are inevitably family diseases, affecting everyone in the family. Treatment must focus on the entire family and treatment continues after the patient dies.

Karl Snepp begins this section with a poignant personal perspective of his adult son's struggle with cancer. In this short piece, he makes three vital points. First, he reminds readers that the illness and death of a child—at *any* age— intimately involves the parents and siblings. Often, especially when there is a spouse and children, parents can be neglected. Second, Snepp recommends that parents be involved, to the degree that is viable, in consultations and decisions regarding the illness. Finally, Snepp advises that parents seek out support such as The Compassionate Friends to reconstruct a life torn asunder by the death of an adult child.

Charles Corr's chapter reaffirms this family focus. From the onset of the disease, all family members live with the illness. Grief then becomes part of the experience as the family copes with a multiplicity of losses throughout the illness such as loss of income, significant roles, health, and even a sense of psychic security. Corr offers a host of suggestions for family members that emphasize the need for ongoing communication and collaborative planning. He recommends the process of reminiscence as an important tool for building a sense of a meaningful life—a critical spiritual need. Corr reiterates a crucial insight: Even in the midst of illness and grief, there remain opportunities for growth.

Kenneth Doka continues this section with a chapter on grief after the death. Doka notes some of the facilitating and complicating factors when an individual dies of cancer. In many ways, this chapter offers a fitting conclusion; he notes that many of the factors previously addressed such as guilt and blame, ethical decisions at the end of life, and the caregiving process not only affect the ways that a patient may die but also influence the family's subsequent grief.

The section concludes with Yvette Colón's personal perspective. Colón describes her mother's bout with cancer. Kastenbaum (1988) once described *vicarious grief* as a form of grief experienced by caregivers as they work with families. To Kastenbaum, the caregiver may be well aware of the likely prognosis even as the patient and family strive to maintain optimism. The caregiver hence has to support that sense of hope even as the caregiver has a clear perspective on where the illness is likely to lead. Colón has a unique perspective and story as she guides her mother through end-of-life care—consciously balancing the skill and knowledge of an oncology social worker with the love of a devoted daughter. Colón's story is a vivid reminder of how much this topic touches us, both personally and professionally.

REFERENCE

Kastenbaum, R. (1988). Vicarious grief as an intergenerational phenomenon. *Death Studies, 12,* 447–453.

Personal Perspective:
He Was Still Our Child

Karl Snepp

From the beginning, our involvement as parents in Dave's illness seemed natural. Never mind that he was an adult with a very responsible job formulating the geometry of wing design for commercial jetliners, comfortably living on his own at the opposite end of the country from our Pennsylvania home. He was our *son*, our *child*, and *parents take care of their children*. So when he told us he had discovered a lump on his neck and probably was going to require surgery, Sue and I quickly arranged to fly to Seattle. It was an instinctive parental reaction.

The "lump" turned out to be medullary thyroid cancer, and for the next 9 years, through the ebbing and flowing of this defiant disease and its final, inexorable surge that took Dave's life, we parented. But we parented differently than we would have if Dave had been younger and living at home.

When a young child has a chronic life-limiting illness, it is important that parents include the child in the treatment decision-making process to the extent the child's maturity allows. In our case, the roles were reversed: Dave, our "child," included *us*, the parents—and Karen, his younger sister by 2 years—in *his* treatment decisions.

For many months at a stretch during Dave's illness, he both appeared and felt healthy. He loved his work and led an active life, pursuing hobbies of photography, biking, and exploring the spectacular Pacific Northwest. But also during those 9 years, Dave underwent two major surgeries, several minor procedures, two courses of radiation, and a discouraging attempt at chemotherapy. Each time his beautiful life was jerked back to the reality of his cancer and it was once again time to plan a next step, he huddled with us before making his decision. We helped him research recent medical developments. We collaborated with him in arranging consultations with specialists in other cities. We were his staff.

When Dave's cancer began to seriously limit his mobility, it became obvious that he would lose much of his self-sufficiency. To put off as long as possible the need to be confined to bed, he was fitted with a halo brace: a cage-like structure to support his head and immobilize his cancer-weakened cervical vertebrae. It would enable him to live at home, walk short distances, and go on wheelchair outings—all, of course, with the aid of a helper.

Sue became that helper. The decision was a no-brainer. Dave's home, employer, network of friends, and medical support were in the Seattle area, which had become so much a part of his life. Sue would move in with Dave and be the helper that he needed to have on hand 24/7, and Karen and I would be there as much as our jobs would allow.

Taking their cue from Dave, the clinicians involved in his care readily accepted our parental role. Sue received valuable guidance from the team of palliative care professionals who became regular visitors to Dave's apartment: his nurse, who immediately won his trust by doing her homework on his unusual cancer before they met; the jolly, motherly aide who kept Dave entertained during bath time with the latest stories of her extended family; the occupational therapist, whose husband built a platform to elevate Dave's recliner, making it easier to use. Looking back, I marvel at how adept they all were at meeting our needs as parents without compromising any of their professional obligations to Dave, their adult patient and client.

Dave died at the end of a 3-day holiday weekend that had allowed both Karen and me to be there. Although he had been unconscious most of his final day, we're pretty sure he waited until the last hours of the weekend on purpose. Karen, Sue, and I were holding his hands. It was his final family huddle.

Months later, when we learned of The Compassionate Friends,* the national self-help support organization for families after a child dies, we were not sure it would be for us. Dave was nearly 33 years old when he died—definitely not a child, although we certainly were parents whose child had died. One of TCF's 600-plus local chapters met regularly about 10 minutes from our home, so we gave it a try. We needn't have worried. Our child had died, and regardless of his age, whatever the cause of his death, or how long it had been, we were welcomed with open, understanding arms. It was a lifeline to our new normal.

---

*www.compassionatefriends.org or toll-free (877) 969-0010.

Karl Snepp *and his wife, Sue, became active volunteers with The Compassionate Friends in the years following Dave's death. After Karl's retirement from ARA Services (now Aramark) in Philadelphia, they moved to Tucson, Arizona, and subsequently became leaders of TCF's local chapter there. Both Karl and Sue have served The Compassionate Friends in various other local, regional, and national capacities, including directorship of TCF's Chapter Leadership Training Program during its development and early years. Karl and Sue now live in Redmond, Washington, near their daughter, Karen, enjoying the Pacific Northwest and occasional travel elsewhere—especially to first-round NCAA basketball tournament venues.*

CHAPTER 13

Cancer, Anticipatory Grief, and Anticipatory Mourning

Charles A. Corr

This chapter links together four central concepts: "cancer," the name for a variety of diseases involving malignant cells that proliferate in ways that do harm to the body; "grief," the term for reactions to losses of various types; "mourning," the designation for processes of responding to grief and loss through coping and adaptive strategies; and "anticipation," or expectations about events that have not yet occurred. The goal is to improve understanding and help individuals, family members, and care providers more effectively live with these realities. This chapter is organized into six headings: disease; illness; anticipated losses; grief reactions and anticipatory grief; mourning responses and anticipatory mourning; and opportunities for growth. Two concluding sections offer some suggestions for individuals with cancer and for those who care for them.

DISEASE

As explained elsewhere in this book, there are many different types of cancer. Some are relatively benign while others are far more dangerous. Some develop very gradually while others advance rapidly. Some cancers have distressing side effects while others grow silently for a long time without obvious manifestations. Some cancers can be cured or reversed while others can only be slowed in their progress and still others may not be open to any cure-oriented intervention by the time they are discovered.

Intervention strategies differ for different types of cancers, the point at which they are diagnosed, and the age of an individual. For example, it is often recommended that older males who are diagnosed with prostate cancer should adopt a posture of "watchful waiting" since this cancer develops quite slowly and may never warrant more active intervention. In many—perhaps most—other cases, typical interventions include surgery, radiotherapy, chemotherapy, or some combination of these.

This suggests that the first thing to consider when one is confronted by a diagnosis of cancer is the specific disease and its implications in the life of a particular individual. Knowing as much as possible about this unique situation is the indispensable foundation upon which everything else follows.

ILLNESS

Arthur Frank (2002), himself a person once diagnosed with cancer, recommended that we make a distinction between "disease"—that which is measurable, quantifiable, and objective—and "illness," or "the experience of living through the disease" (p. 13). From this perspective, it is important for every individual diagnosed with cancer to consider how he or she is living with and through this disease. One might ask: Where was I in my life when I received this diagnosis and where am I now?

More specifically, Doka (1993, 2009) has suggested there are at least five possible phases in living with a disease like cancer:

- The *prediagnostic phase* in which there are some initial indicators of disease: Should I ignore them hoping "it" will go away, try to minimize my affective reactions to them, or investigate them and try to seek help of some type?

- The *acute phase* in which I might do things like try to understand the disease, maximize health and lifestyle, foster coping strengths and limit weaknesses, develop strategies to deal with issues created by the disease, arrange for cure-oriented interventions, explore effects of the diagnosis on my sense of self and others, ventilate feelings and fears, and/or incorporate the reality of the diagnosis into my sense of past and future.

- The *chronic phase* of living with the disease in which I might try to manage symptoms and side effects, seek to prevent and manage health crises, manage stress and examine coping, maximize social support and minimize isolation, normalize life, deal with psychological, social, and other concerns, and try to find meaning in suffering, uncertainty, and decline.

- Since cancer does not always lead to death, there may be a *recovery phase* in which I might need to deal with the aftereffects of disease-related events and anxieties about recurrence, reconstruct a new lifestyle, and redefine relationships with caregivers.

- When cancer does lead inexorably to death, the *terminal phase* is a time in which I might need to deal with ongoing challenges from the disease, side effects, and interventions; make decisions about continuing or discontinuing curative interventions or putting more emphasis on palliative care; and prepare for death and saying goodbye.

This schema reminds us that there is almost always some time at our disposal; cancer rarely acts like a sudden death. During that time there are temporal variables involving past, present, and future—things that have already happened, things that are currently happening, and things that are expected to happen. There are also a wide variety of social, cultural, psychological, and personal variables that influence coping with the disease. Above all, there are choices that one can make as one lives through the disease.

ANTICIPATED LOSSES

Most discussions of grief and mourning relate to losses that have already occurred or are currently occurring. Those losses are certainly important. However, our charge is to consider losses that have not yet occurred, but that are expected to occur. This implies that one has received some type of forewarning about the possibility of such losses—some sign that makes one think such losses might occur in the near future.

Forewarning is a necessary but not sufficient condition for attending and taking some action relating to a possible loss. I might, for example, ignore the warning, not give it much credence, assume that it applies to others but not to me, or believe that it will only apply to me at some relatively distant point in the future.

When I do take the warning to heart, however, my attention is likely to focus on the losses I anticipate. For example, when one man was told of his diagnosis of cancer, he interpreted that to mean his death was imminent. When he shared that interpretation with his wife, she found it difficult to believe and checked with the physician. She was able to tell her husband that his interpretation was wrong. What this man learned was that his expectations were not realistic. In other words, expectations about anticipated losses may be more or less accurate. An individual may have misunderstood the warning associated with a diagnosis and may have come to think that a particular loss is to be expected when in fact it is not at all likely. Fears and anxieties generated by the diagnosis may have led someone to imagine terrifying possibilities that are beyond the realm of any reasonable expectation. That is one reason why providers should share truthful information with those in their care no matter how dire that information may seem, since an individual's imagination may lead to expectations that are far worse than what can reasonably be expected to occur.

Still, the main point is that my anticipations of losses that are yet to come, however accurate or inaccurate they may be, are part of my overall journey with a disease like cancer.

GRIEF REACTIONS AND ANTICIPATORY GRIEF

Grief, as noted earlier, is the term used to indicate one's reactions to loss (Rando, 1984, 1993). When a person experiences a significant loss, it is expected that he or she would react in some way. Not to react in any manner would be surprising. It would suggest that the loss was insignificant to the individual, that the relationship was complicated in ways that set it apart from the ordinary, or that the individual is somehow suppressing or hiding his or her reactions to the loss. So let's work under the assumption that in ordinary, uncomplicated situations, individuals can be expected to react when a significant loss occurs in their lives and let's agree to call that reaction "grief."

The losses to which one is reacting may be of many different types. They may be what are called primary losses, such as the ending or termination of a relationship, or secondary losses, such as those that follow upon a primary loss. They may relate to a diagnosis such as cancer, to an attachment such as that to a spouse or partner, to a cherished object or social status, or to the possibility of death. Here, we focus on reactions to losses that are anticipated but have not yet actually taken place.

For example, following his diagnosis of cancer, John and his wife, Kate, found themselves thinking about the possible financial burdens involved with John's treatment. They became anxious about what treatment would mean for their budget and especially about the possibility that John might lose his job if he became weaker and his sick leave ran out. John found it hard to sleep as he pondered these thoughts while Kate experienced unexpected bouts of crying. All of these reactions to the losses that this couple might experience are perfectly understandable, even if the anticipated losses never actually arise.

Anyone who has personally experienced grief or who has encountered a grieving person will know that grief reactions to any loss can be experienced and expressed in numerous ways. Worden (2009) describes normal grief reactions in four general categories:

- *Feelings*, such as sadness, anger, guilt and self-reproach, anxiety, loneliness, fatigue, helplessness, shock, yearning or pining, emancipation, relief, and numbness
- *Physical sensations*, such as hollowness in the stomach, tightness in the chest or throat, aching arms, oversensitivity to noise, a sense of depersonalization, shortness of breath, muscle weakness, lack of energy, and dry mouth
- *Cognitions*, such as disbelief, confusion, preoccupation, a sense of presence of the deceased, and paranormal experiences ("hallucinations")
- *Behaviors*, such as sleep or appetite disturbances, absentmindedness, social withdrawal, dreams of the deceased, avoiding reminders of the deceased, searching and calling out, sighing, restless hyperactivity, crying, visiting places or carrying objects that remind the survivor of the deceased, and treasuring objects that belonged to the deceased

Worden's categories include *social dimensions* of grief under behaviors, although it might be better to identify them separately. S*piritual dimensions* of grief should also be mentioned since they are so common in loss situations. Spiritual dimensions of grief might include hostility toward God or a higher power, on the one hand, or calling upon one's religious convictions to buffer or incorporate the loss, on the other hand.

The most important thing to say about this broad description of grief is that any or all of these reactions—experienced inwardly or outwardly, expressed privately or publicly—are almost always healthy, normal, and appropriate. Unhealthy, complicated, or prolonged grief reactions do occur as a disorder in a small percentage of people. Still, for most individuals who have not previously experienced significant loss in their lives, grief reactions may be *unusual*, but they are not *abnormal*. They are signs or manifestations of the distress associated with loss, not symptoms of disease. Grief is a "dis-ease," a discomforting disturbance of everyday equilibrium, but it is not a "disease" in the sense of a sickness or unhealthy condition of mind or body. Any human reaction can, of course, be carried to an unhealthy extreme, but ordinary, uncomplicated grief is an understandable and fitting reaction to a significant loss in one's life.

One other point to notice is that grief reactions are individual—unique to each particular loss and each bereaved person. The same individual is likely to react in different ways to different losses; different individuals are likely to react in different ways to the same loss. John and Kate each had their own grief reactions to their anticipated losses. For this reason, apart from extreme grief reactions that may lead to harm to oneself or others, one person's grief should not be used as a standard to evaluate the grief of others.

In terms of the focus of this chapter, when an individual has come to anticipate a loss, it is not surprising for such an individual to react to his or her expectations and thus to experience grief reactions in relation to those expectations. As part of the individual's psychic world, the anticipation is sufficient to generate a grief reaction of one type or another. For example, one might experience anticipatory grief in advance of the death of a loved one even though that death has not yet occurred. Here one would be experiencing grief reactions because one expects the loved one to die. Note again that the validity of the person's expectation is not relevant. Simply taking the expectation as real might be enough to generate grief reactions. In principle, anticipatory grief refers to grief experiences that take place prior to but in relation to a significant loss that is expected to take place but has not yet occurred (Rando, 1986).

MOURNING RESPONSES AND ANTICIPATORY MOURNING

Worden (2009) recently wrote, "I am using the term 'mourning' to indicate the process that occurs after a loss, while 'grief' refers to the personal experience of the loss" (p. 37). That at least draws a distinction between the terms *grief* and *mourning*. But perhaps it would be more accurate to think of *mourning* as the term for efforts to cope with loss and grief, on the one hand, and efforts to adapt to and develop healthy ways to live in a new world, on the other hand (see, e.g., Corr, Nabe, & Corr, 2009; Rando, 1984, 1993). If so, mourning has two complementary forms or aspects: as Stroebe and Schut (1999) point out in their dual process model, mourning or coping with loss involves a dynamic oscillation between "loss-oriented processes" and "restoration-oriented processes." That is, mourning takes into account both (1) the loss (here one that is anticipated or expected to occur) and its associated grief reactions; and (2) the new world that will arise if and when the loss occurs, together with the "new normals" that the individual will need to develop to healthily live in that new world. As a result, mourning can encompass both internal, private, or intrapersonal processes, and external, public, or interpersonal processes.

The important point is to focus not just on grief reactions, but on the larger and in some ways more important processes of mourning. This is because, as Shneidman (1980/1995) once wrote, "Mourning is one of the most profound human experiences that it is possible to have....The deep capacity to weep for the loss of a loved one and to continue to treasure the memory of that loss is one of our noblest human traits" (p. 179).

Just as post-death mourning focuses on losses that have already taken place, anticipatory mourning focuses on anticipated losses and the grief reactions linked to those losses (Rando, 2000). In the example of John and Kate mentioned above, the two of them talked together about what they would do if their anticipated losses came to pass, and they were careful to pledge to honor each other's anticipatory grief reactions. In addition, in order to improve their financial situation, John sold off some property he had inherited and Kate began a course at the local community college in case she would need to go back to work.

In another situation, after he was diagnosed with cancer, Orville Kelly found himself being subjected to stigma and discrimination. He might have known that people often behave this way when they do not understand certain diseases and are frightened by them. In the past, this happened to individuals with leprosy or tuberculosis; in our time, cancer and HIV/AIDS are diseases that have been overlaid with external burdens. Sontag (1978) called this process "illness as metaphor." When Kelly recognized how unfairly he was being treated as a result of social metaphors, he fought back by adopting "Make today count" as the maxim on which he would base the remainder of his life. He also wrote a book (Kelly, 1975) and founded an organization with the same name to help others in similar situations.

Once again, Arthur Frank (2002) is a useful guide in reminding us that we have opportunities even when we are coping with difficult diseases and mourning anticipated losses:

> The word "victim" is a half-truth. We may be victims of disease, but we are not victims of illness....Choice becomes possible when we shift the perspective from the disease to the illness. Because we can choose how we experience illness, we can be more than victims.... But choices are limited....We can choose only from what is available. We are not victims of circumstances, but circumstances limit our choices. . . . (p. 138)

OPPORTUNITIES FOR GROWTH

Time spent living with cancer is both pressured and precious. It is *pressured* because of all the demands and stresses that the disease has imposed and will continue to impose. Persons with cancer may already have made changes in their daily routines and have found themselves interacting with unfamiliar health systems or care providers. They may be experiencing loss of energy, difficult symptoms, or limitations in what they can do. Nevertheless, this is also a very *precious* time in their lives. It is a time they will never have again. In this precious time, such persons can make choices that will affect the quality of their lives now and in the near future. These choices can also affect the lives of others around them in important ways, both now and well into the future. They can make choices—within limits—about how they use this time currently available to them.

A person living with cancer still has the possibility of opportunities for growth in his or her life. The diagnosis can lead the person to reflect on his or her life and its meaning. People often speak of "unfinished business" in circumstances like these. This refers both to aspects of personal or spiritual relationships and to various practical matters. For the former, one might ask questions like: Am I content or "at peace" with all aspects of my life? Am I content with my relations with people I love or can I improve them? Are there things I might want to do or say to people whom I love? Can I arrange to spend time with such people, perhaps to share my values with them or to arrange to leave positive legacies with them? Have I been able to find or construct meaning in my life, or perhaps can I engage in such a project as I live in this precious time? Why not do those things now?

From a more practical standpoint, other questions might arise like: Have I undertaken or completed projects I value? Have I filled out an advance directive to govern the care I want to receive if I become unable to take part in decision making now or at the end of my life? Advance directives include living wills and durable powers of attorney in healthcare matters (sometimes called healthcare proxies) that appoint an agent or substitute decision maker to determine how things should go.

I might also want to be sure my estate is in order and that arrangements have been made to ensure that the rituals following my death will reflect the values and wishes I believe have characterized my life. Advance planning of funeral or memorial services can relieve family members and loved ones as much as possible of the burden of these responsibilities after death. An updated will can ensure that my property will be distributed as I wish.

Living with a disease like cancer may lead a person to anticipate losses and to grieve and mourn those expected losses. But reflecting on one's illness can also lead to identifying new challenges and new opportunities in one's life. A person can take up those challenges and opportunities or decline to do so. The point is that only that particular person can decide what to do.

Some Suggestions for Individuals Who Are Living with Cancer, Anticipatory Grief, and Anticipatory Mourning

Socrates once said that "the unexamined life is not worth living." For Socrates, the key to developing an examined life is to "know thyself." This theme can help us develop some practical lessons for individuals with cancer.

- Begin by knowing as much as you reasonably can about your disease. Seek out information from your oncologist, your family physician, other healthcare providers, articles, books, the Internet, and other reliable sources. The more you know about the specifics of your particular form of cancer, the better you will be prepared to make the decisions you need to make.

- Reflect on what Arthur Frank called your "illness" or how you are living with this disease. How have you been living with this disease? How are you currently living with it? How might you live with it in the future and during the above phases identified by Doka? As the well-known Serenity Prayer advises, we need to have the wisdom to distinguish between the things we can change and things we cannot; the courage to change the things that should be changed; and the grace to accept with serenity the things that cannot be changed (Sifton, 2003).

- Scrutinize the losses you anticipate for the near future and the choices you have made about your illness. Evaluate carefully the forewarnings you have received as well as your suspicions, premonitions, or expectations about anticipated losses. Be realistic in this process so that you don't mislead, unduly burden, or even torture yourself with unrealistic expectations.

- Examine your grief reactions to those anticipated losses, taking into account the full range of possible reactions—including physical, psychological (affective and cognitive), behavioral, social, and spiritual dimensions. This is another way of knowing yourself, in a way particularly linked to your disease, illness, and anticipated losses. Recognize the legitimacy of your own grief experiences; don't impose upon yourself some external schema or theory about grief or someone else's advice about how you should be grieving. This is your life and your journey with loss and grief—not theirs. Recognize that your grief reactions may change in different contexts and may differ at different points as you live with your disease.

- Consider how you are mourning or coping with your disease, your anticipated losses, and your grief reactions to those losses. Coping with these realities and expectations and adapting to the new world in which you find yourself is the heart of anticipatory mourning. It is also the essence of the advice we are given in both the Serenity Prayer and in the "Make Today Count" maxim.
- Remain open to opportunities for growth. As long as you are alive and alert, you can decide how to live your life and how to make things better for yourself and those you love.

SOME SUGGESTIONS FOR FAMILY MEMBERS AND CARE PROVIDERS

Insofar as family members and care providers are living with a person who has cancer, they too may be experiencing anticipatory grief and anticipatory mourning. If so, then many of the suggestions in the previous section may apply to them with appropriate modifications. Beyond that, in their roles as helpers it may be useful for them to

- Remember that you are a different individual than the person with cancer. This suggests the great value of listening versus talking, as well as silence at appropriate times. Be cautious in supplying answers that you find meaningful for yourself. If asked, offer perspectives in light of your life experiences, not as absolute truths for everyone.
- Recognize that the person for whom you are providing care is coping with serious challenges (including anticipated losses) and tasks that he or she must carry out for him- or herself. Be authentically present by attending to that person, his or her tasks, and what he or she wants from you.
- Respect the meaning and values of the person for whom you are providing care, including that person's anticipatory grief reactions and anticipatory mourning processes. Avoid being judgmental.

- Reinforce the person's decision-making capacity and support his or her actual decisions. Help the person clarify his or her decisions and choices, and be an advocate for their realization.
- Reminisce with the person about his or her life and meaning. Elicit stories from the person about his or her life experiences. Make available activities and materials that are important to the person and that help in the development of meaning (adapted from Corr, Nabe, & Corr, 2009, p. 168).

Charles A. Corr, *PhD, CT, is a member of the board of directors of the Suncoast Institute, an affiliate of Suncoast Hospice, the ChiPPS (Children's Project on Palliative/Hospice Services) Leadership Advisory Council of the National Hospice and Palliative Care Organization, the Executive Committee of the National Donor Family Council, the Association for Death Education and Counseling, and the International Work Group on Death, Dying, and Bereavement (Chairperson, 1989–93). He is also professor emeritus, Southern Illinois University, Edwardsville. Dr. Corr's publications in the field of death, dying, and bereavement include three dozen books and booklets, along with more than 100 chapters and articles in professional publications. His most recent publication is the sixth edition of* Death and Dying, Life and Living *(Belmont, CA: Wadsworth, 2009), co-authored with Clyde M. Nabe and Donna M. Corr.*

REFERENCES

Corr, C. A., Nabe, C. M., & Corr, D. M. (2009). *Death and dying, life and living* (6th ed.). Belmont, CA: Wadsworth.

Doka, K. J. (1993). *Living with life-threatening illness: A guide for patients, families, and caregivers.* Lexington, MA: Lexington Books.

Doka, K. J. (2009). *Counseling individuals with life-threatening illness.* New York: Springer Publishing.

Frank, A. (2002). *At the will of the body: Reflections on illness* (originally 1991; now with a new Afterword). Boston: Houghton Mifflin.

Kelly, O. (1975). *Make today count.* New York: Delacorte Press.

Rando, T. A. (1984). *Grief, dying, and death: Clinical interventions for caregivers.* Champaign, IL: Research Press.

Rando, T. A. (1986). *Loss and anticipatory grief.* Lexington, MA: Lexington Books.

Rando, T. A. (1993). *Treatment of complicated mourning.* Champaign, IL: Research Press.

Rando, T. A. (2000). *Clinical dimensions of anticipatory mourning: Theory and practice in working with the dying, their loved ones, and their caregivers.* Champaign, IL: Research Press.

Shneidman, E. S. (1980/1995). *Voices of death.* New York: Harper & Row/ Kodansha International.

Sifton, E. (2003). *The serenity prayer: Faith and politics in time of peace and war.* New York: Norton.

Sontag, S. (1978). *Illness as metaphor.* New York: Farrar, Straus & Giroux.

Stroebe, M., & Schut, H. (1999). The dual process model of coping with bereavement: Rationale and description. *Death Studies, 23,* 197–224.

Worden, J. W. (2009). *Grief counseling and grief therapy: A handbook for the mental health practitioner* (4th ed.). New York: Springer Publishing.

Grief After a Death From Cancer

Kenneth J. Doka

A s we know, cancer is not a single disease. There are over 150 different types of cancer. Some are relatively treatable and boast high cure rates while others are more lethal. Some, such as lung cancer, are associated with habits or behaviors and may cause a sense of guilt, blame, and opprobrium. Other forms of cancer may be highly disfiguring, create considerable suffering, or cause personality changes. Such conditions can create ambivalence on the part of survivors that can complicate grief. Moreover, the many decisions associated with a cancer diagnosis—from diagnosis and treatment to end-of-life care and decisions—can generate other complicating factors for survivors' grief. Different forms of cancer can create very distinct issues that haunt families after a cancer death.

This chapter begins by exploring in more depth these complicating factors, offering strategies for health and bereavement professionals as they deal with families. However, it also notes the unique role that health professionals may have in treating cancer. Since cancer is often a prolonged illness, professionals may develop relationships with patients and families that span years. These professionals may also experience grief when a patient dies. This issue also needs to be explored in this chapter.

COMPLICATING FACTORS IN CANCER DEATHS

Prolonged Illness and Grief

Early research (Rando, 1983; Sanders, 1983) indicated that while sudden loss raises complications for grief, so does prolonged illness. There are a number of reasons for this. In prolonged illness, there is often the perception that the ill person suffered a great deal through the illness experience. In addition, there is likely to be considerable disfigurement. In many cancers, for example, patients may waste away to a seemingly skeletal version of a former self. Other cancers may cause unsightly tumors or disfigure a patient's face or neck. Other times, there may be physical residues of the treatment: hair loss, amputations, bloating, or scarring. Such disfigurement can exacerbate perceptions that the patient is suffering. Moreover, disfiguring illnesses add to a sense of ambivalence (Doka, 1997). As the illness disfigures the patient, family and significant others may find themselves physically repulsed by the patient's appearance even as they continue to love and care for the person. These mixed feelings can generate a strong sense of guilt when the patient dies. Both guilt and ambivalence are associated with complicated grief (Rando, 1993; Doka, 1997).

In certain forms of cancer, such a brain tumor, there can be considerable personality changes and mental deterioration. This can result from both the disease process or as a side effect of treatment. In and of itself, these changes create an additional sense of loss—a form of psychosocial loss. That is, the persona of the patient is so changed that family and friends grieve the person who once was. This can even be the case when changes are positive. For example, in one case, a patient with a history of alcohol abuse ceased drinking as he underwent chemotherapy. After his death, his wife described the time of his illness as one of the best in their marriage. She felt cheated of all the time that was missed throughout their married life because of his alcoholism. In other cases, negative changes in personality may lead to increased ambivalence and complicate memories of the person who died as well as the sense of the relationship, thus complicating grief.

Blame, Guilt, and Disenfranchised Grief

Issues of guilt and blame also can complicate grief when someone dies of cancer. There can be multiple sources of guilt. Some forms of cancer are identified with lifestyle factors such as tobacco use. While studies have shown mixed results in the extent to which even smokers see their tobacco use as responsible for cancer (Bertero, Vanhanen, & Appelin, 2008; Mumma & McCorkle, 1983), other studies have indicated that persons with lung cancer recognize that the stigma of smoking is associated with their illness and believe the stigma has lessened support (Chapple, Ziebland, & McPherson, 2004; Faller, Schilling, & Lang, 1995). The perception that the individual shares responsibility for his or her illness may not only lessen support during the course of the illness, but also disenfranchise the grief of survivors (Doka, 2002).

Even where there is no perceived link to causation, there may be other sources of guilt. Since mortality rates vary among types of cancers and prognosis is often uncertain, there may be a perception that the patient did not fight hard enough to survive (Berckman & Austin, 1993). Given that cancer is an extended illness, that early detection enhances survival in many forms of cancer, and that there are often choices of treatment modalities, there are numerous opportunities for surviving family members to reassess choices and decisions made throughout the course of the illness. Blame and guilt may result, centered perhaps on the patient, health professionals who were perceived to have been slow to respond or treat, or surviving family members including oneself. In summary, issues of guilt and blame should always be evaluated in grief assessments.

Ethical Decisions at the End of Life

Ethical decisions made at the end of life also can complicate grief (Doka, 2005). The individual or family making the decision can be torn between a desire to end suffering and a continued quest to retain hope even in the midst of impending death. Individuals or family members may experience conflict between following their own beliefs and honoring the expressed wishes of the deceased.

Sometimes the conflict can be between family members. Since one person within the family system generally holds the health proxy, there may be discord as other family members question decisions that have been made. These end-of-life decisions can create family conflicts or revive family disputes. Such disagreements can limit subsequent support while generating concurrent crises such as family fights that complicate the grief process.

The manner of death, too, may complicate subsequent grief. The decision to terminate life support may not ensure an easy death. Family members may even interpret or misinterpret the final actions of the dying person as evidence of pain and distress. Even when the death does not occur with signs of evident distress, families may be uncomfortable with the circumstances surrounding the death. For example, it is generally believed that neither artificial feeding nor hydration is necessarily palliative. Yet, decision makers or other family members may still perceive that the patient died thirsty or hungry, complicating grief. On the other hand, decisions to continue treatment may lead families to believe that the patient needlessly suffered. Family decision makers then may wish they acted to ease such suffering.

Two final points should be made in this section. End-of-life decisions are generally made in a context of interaction and communication with medical staff. Mixed messages, poor communication, staff disapproval of decisions, and isolation can exacerbate the decision-making process, increasing both individual distress as well as familial conflict.

Second, these decisions need not necessarily complicate the grieving process. Active involvement in the decision-making process may give surviving family members a sense of control in an otherwise uncontrollable time and may result in a sense that their actions contributed to an eased death for their loved one.

Loss, Grief, and the Caregiving Experience

The caregiving experience should be explored as well. Grief is inherent in caregiving, as caregivers must relinquish time, roles, and independence as they assume the role of caregiver. At the time of death, the caregiving experience may both facilitate and complicate grief. Prolonged illness, especially when it involves caregiving responsibilities, allows surviving family members the opportunity and insight to see the physical deterioration of the patient. Thus, there is less sense of shock at the time of death.

Moreover, prolonged illness does give individuals opportunity to finish business—to say goodbye, talk over past issues, and possibly resolve conflict. And the very experience of caregiving can be a demonstration of love that may be perceived as atoning for prior conflicts and difficulties.

While there are aspects that facilitate grief, other factors complicate it. Prolonged illness and caregiving are both stressful. This affects grief in at least four ways. First, the cumulative effects of prolonged stress from the illness and caregiving are draining, sapping the ability to respond to yet another series of stressful events necessitated by the loss. In such cases, it is not unusual for caregivers to experience a range of reactions that might complicate grief such as guilt or even relief to be freed from the incessant demands of caregiving, arousing yet more guilt.

Second, these effects may be experienced throughout the social network, limiting opportunities for support. Third, an extensive period of caregiving can isolate caregivers from their traditional support networks. These networks might be dissipated by the time of the patient's death, limiting social support. Fourth, the stressful context of caregiving can fray relationships, creating or exacerbating conflicts between caregivers or with the dying person that may need to be later addressed (see Doka, 2001). It is no surprise that caregiving for family members dying of cancer has been associated with high levels of distress (Tomarken et al., 2008).

When a Child Dies

Though the death rates for children and adolescents in developed societies tend to be low, cancer remains a major cause of nontraumatic death in childhood and adolescence. The death of a child is inherently complicated as it challenges parental suppositions that they will predecease their child, hence challenging their assumptive world (Rando, 1993). Moreover, the death of a child creates widespread grieving affecting surviving siblings and grandparents. Grandparents are often disenfranchised in their grief—expected to support the parents despite their own significant sense of loss (Nehari, Grebler, & Toren, 2007). When an adult child dies, surviving parents may be disenfranchised. In these cases, the parental assumption still remains that their child will remain alive through the parents' lives. When an adult child dies, the focus of support often is on the surviving spouse and children.

INTERVENTIONS AFTER A CANCER DEATH

As the Patient Approaches Death: Needs and Interventions[1]

When families and intimate networks are approaching the imminent death of a cancer patient, they may need the following help as they deal with their ongoing needs.

Dealing with affect. Families may struggle with a series of ambivalent emotions as death approaches. They may feel relief and subsequent guilt as they anticipate the end of caregiving. They may struggle with all the emotions of grief. They will need opportunities for validation and information. In the beginning of the terminal phase, families may need to understand their options when care is palliative. These options may include varied bridge programs, hospice, or palliative care programs. As death approaches, families may need to be informed about what will occur as the patient actively dies. Such information may inform any ethical choices at the end of life.

Balancing demands. For many caregivers, responsibilities and demands may increase. Caregivers may need assistance at this time prioritizing and balancing

---

1 Material from this section is drawn from Doka (2001).

the varied responsibilities they face as well as finding and accepting support from formal and informal networks.

Interacting with the patient in meaningful ways. Even as the patient's life ebbs, family members can still communicate in meaningful ways. If the patient is conscious, there are varied opportunities for life review and offering legacies. For example, in living eulogies, family and friends are invited to share their memories with the patient prior to death. With ethical wills, patients address the values they would like to pass on to their intimate network. Dignity therapy trains volunteers to work with patients, constructing a bound life story of the patient that is shared prior to death and then presented to the family. Research has indicated that these meaning-centered approaches have value for patients and families (McClement et al., 2007). Even when the patient is comatose, family members can be encouraged to continue to touch and communicate with the patient as well as to engage in ritual and spiritual activities such as prayer or readings.

Preparing for death. Families may need to focus on what they will need to do as death approaches. Have they made plans for a funeral? Are legal documents such as advance directives in order? What are personal acts that they may need to do prior to a patient's death? Is there a particular way that they need to say goodbye?

Professionals can assist family caregivers in a number of ways here. First, family members will need information on what to expect as death occurs. They may need to review advance directives. As stated earlier, it may be critical here to review decisions. For example, family members may need to be reminded that feeding tubes or hydration may cause additional discomfort at the end of life. Such information at this time may eliminate potential conflicts and mitigate later distress over actions. Second, family caregivers may need to review and rehearse final actions. As death approaches, for example, they should know who to call and what they need to do.

When Death Occurs

At the time of death, a number of interventions will assist caregivers:

Allow time alone. Do not rush removal of the body. Remember that the family may need time alone to say goodbye.

Empower ritual. The moment of death is a sacred time. Offer them options for a ritual. Perhaps they would wish to light a candle, say a prayer, or find another meaningful way to address the moment.

Allow grief. It is appropriate at this moment for families to express their grief. Do not and—as much as is in one's power—do not let others inhibit that expression.

Help with the details. Families may be confused and disoriented at this time. They may value assistance in calling the funeral home and informing others (Doka, 2001).

After the Death[2]

Validate expressions of grief. Validation is an essential aspect of grief support. Validation means that individuals' experience of grief is listened to, understood, accepted, and explained as a valid response to the loss. No expressions of grief are inappropriate. Responses such as "You shouldn't feel guilty" or "How can you be upset after all your years together" are common but serve to deny and invalidate grief. Rather, patients and caregivers need to have these experiences of loss and expressions of grief acknowledged. This gives space for individuals to explore their many reactions to their experience. This is critical.

Help families deal with the affective issues aroused by the loss. As stated earlier, patients and their networks often lack opportunities to ventilate the emotions aroused by the situation. When the patient was alive, family and friends may feel disloyal, unfeeling, or inhibited in expressing emotion. Counselors should encourage emotional expression, identify and validate the emotional responses that clients experience, and explore strategies for coping with these emotions. It is critical that counselors recognize the broad range of ways in which clients may achieve emotional release. For some, ventilating by crying can be helpful; for others, emotional energy can be expressed in activity or cognition (Martin & Doka, 1999).

Help individuals recognize and respond to the changes in their own lives. An individual who experiences loss is likely to experience a series of secondary losses that spring from the initial loss. Sometimes this may even be a relationship with a professional caregiver. It is not unusual in a cancer death for families to bond with a range of health professionals including secretaries, technicians,

---

2 Worden (2009), Humphrey (2009), and Rando (1993) offer excellent resources for grief counselors.

and aides. Families may need opportunities to recognize the contributions of such individuals to their loved one's care. Many times helping persons to acknowledge these changes can be beneficial. Simply asking, "In what ways has your own life changed since...?" allows individuals to enumerate these losses. Sometimes family members themselves will be surprised at the extent to which their lives have changed. Having identified the losses, individuals can then develop strategies for coping with them, perhaps regaining some of what was lost (possibly in modified form) and mourning the loss of what cannot be salvaged.

Explore methods of coping. Coping can be defined as the "constantly changing cognitive and behavioral efforts to manage specific external and/or internal demands that are appraised as passing or exceeding the resources of the person" (Lazarus & Folkman, 1984, p. 141). Coping strategies can be diverse: Some are helpful (such as reframing thoughts or sharing emotions with others). Because the conditions surrounding loss can create periods of sustained stress, counselors will find it useful to explore individuals' coping strategies. In this exploration, coping strengths can be identified and encouraged. Unhelpful coping strategies can also be identified and clients can then assess alternative strategies. Among the issues that might arise in a discussion of coping strategies are concerns about support. One key coping skill is utilizing one's support system effectively. Asking individuals to identify and assess their informal support systems can be useful in many ways. It can reinforce the idea that there are others to whom they may turn. It can lead to discussions about who has or has not been forthcoming, allowing the assessment of "surprises"—that is, individuals who did not come through as expected or those who provided unexpected support. This discussion can identify barriers to support, such as a reluctance to use or seek support.

Review decisions made in the course of the illness. From the decision to seek treatment, there are numerous decisions in cancer care. Should this mole or lump be examined? Should one try surgery or chemotherapy? Should one enter an experimental protocol? Should one continue treatment or accept that care is now palliative? What decisions should be made as death nears? These are examples of some of the questions encountered throughout the course of cancer therapy. After the death of a patient, family members may need to reexamine the choices made to be assured that they acted wisely with the information they knew at the time.

Reinforce a sense of connection to the person who died. Individuals retain a connection with the person even after that person's death. After a prolonged illness, surviving family members and others may struggle with that sense of connection. They can be overwhelmed with images or behaviors experienced throughout the illness. Counselors can help review the person's life and use expressive approaches such as photographs to help revive memories and images prior to the disease.

Explore spiritual issues raised by the patient's condition. Sometimes, individuals may experience a shattering of assumptions—their beliefs about the nature of the world or the future—which can give rise to a profound spiritual struggle. Again, counselors can validate this struggle, provide space to explore the spiritual issues raised by the illness, and allow clients to assess the ways in which they can effectively utilize their beliefs, rituals, and faith communities.

Counselors may employ many resources as they assist individuals in dealing with losses. Support groups, for example, can offer respite, validation, suggestions for coping, and hope. In many of the same ways, bibliotherapy, or the use of books or self-help literature, can be helpful. Like groups, it can offer validation, help, and suggestions for coping. And it is available whenever an individual needs support and comfort.

Rituals, too, are helpful. Funerals and memorial services that are inclusive, personal, and participatory can allow ventilation of grief reactions, empower a sense of community and social support, stimulate recollections of the deceased, offer structure at a difficult time, provide spiritual succor, and bring mourners together. Therapeutic rituals can be developed throughout the grieving process to reaffirm a continuing bond, mark transitions within the grieving process, affirm the life of the deceased, and finish any unfinished business (Martin and Doka, 1999).

Formal Caregivers and Grief [3]

While healthcare professionals in the past were expected to keep an emotional distance from their patients (Vachon, 1987; Lev, 1989; Figley, 1995), this was difficult to do in practice. Fulton (1987), for example, applied the lessons of the Stockholm syndrome to the health professional-patient relationship. The

---

3 Material here is drawn from Doka (2005).

Stockholm syndrome, which emerged from a study of the relationships between hostages and captors, emphasized that often captors and hostages developed an intense and mutually productive bond. Fulton viewed the phenomenon as broader than that of hostage taking. To Fulton, the underlying process was more inclusive; persons tend to bond quickly in crises. Healthcare workers and other formal caregivers are often involved in intense crises situations that can result in forging a strong bond. Thus when a health professional develops a strong bond with a particular patient, the death of that patient then generates grief. Naturally this bond is individual. Not every caregiver becomes so bonded to each of his or her patients all the time. Yet, certain losses may provoke a strong grief reaction. Papadatou (2000) notes that even beyond the loss of an individual patient, staff may experience additional losses.

This is particularly true in cancer. Treatments often take place over years. Staff, including a range of technicians, may interact with patients and families over years—sharing both the triumphs and disappointments that arise through the course of the disease. When a patient dies, such staff may lose not only a relationship with a patient but with the family as well, exacerbating feelings of loss. The very nature of cancer treatment exacerbates a phenomenon of vicarious grief (Kastenbaum, 1988). Health professionals may have to publicly share the patient and family's optimism while understanding the likely prognosis; in effect, grieving for the family.

Papadatou (2000) also described other factors that contribute to a health professional's sense of loss. Staff may experience a loss of their own unmet goals or expectations regarding the patient. They may have wished to do something else such as additional treatment or perhaps an act of kindness prior to the death. For example, in one case a nurse's sorrow was compounded because her young patient died before she had the opportunity to bake him a promised treat. There may also be a loss of self as the professional confronts his or her own mortality. Staff may experience a reminder of past or anticipated personal losses and their own assumptions or beliefs may be challenged as the patient dies.

There may be factors that complicate the response to death. As patients face the end of life, family members may make decisions that are contrary to the health professional's ethical stance. In some cases, such professionals may have little if any role in such deliberations, intensifying a sense of powerlessness that can affect subsequent grief reactions (Doka, 2005).

This grief can be manifested in many ways including anger, anxiety, powerlessness, hopelessness, sadness, or guilt. Staff can feel they are on emotional roller coaster and become emotionally depleted or depressed. They can become preoccupied with the disease or trauma, perhaps constantly fearing that they or someone they love will have a similar experience or defensively become unfocused, rigid, or apathetic. They may question their beliefs or sense of purpose, or become skeptical. Health professionals may even experience physical manifestations of stress such as aches and pains, sleeping and eating difficulties, or other medical maladies (Figley, 1995).

This grief may affect their relations with others. Staff members may seem angry and impatient. They may withdraw from others, become distrustful, overprotective, or hypervigilant. Such grief even may affect the work environment, lowering morale and contributing to staff turnover (Figley, 1995; Papatadou, 2000).

While the experience of professional grief is similar to other types of losses, Papatadou (2000) reminds us of a major difference in process. Because of the ongoing nature of the work, health professionals have to simultaneously oscillate between containing their grief and experiencing that grief. If staff members fail to contain their grief, they can become overwhelmed by constant loss and be unable to function within their position. However, if professionals constantly contain their grief, eventually this will inhibit contact with their patients. They will gradually dehumanize the person whom they serve. Only by fluctuating between these two processes, Papadatou (2000) posits, can healthcare staff maintain both their effectiveness and humanity.

As noted throughout this chapter, formal caregivers will need to confront their own grief. Both Vachon (1987) and Papadatou (2000) found that both individual and organizational factors influenced adjustment to the effects of cumulative losses, mitigating compassion fatigue. Individuals benefited from effective lifestyle management. Their grief, too, was facilitated by their own ability to validate their own grief and to find their own spiritual center.

Organizational factors also were critical. Organizations assisted health professionals when they acknowledged and supported their grief in such ways as offering education about professional grief, support groups, effective and caring supervision, and rituals where professional caregivers could acknowledge loss.

CONCLUSION

Grief, then, is an inherent part of the cancer experience. It begins at the time of diagnosis, if not even earlier with the anxieties generated from the early yet undiagnosed symptoms. This grief continues even after the death, affecting not only family and friends, but also the health professionals who become part of that intimate network. This grief needs to be acknowledged and treated as surely as the disease.

REFERENCES

Berckman, K. L., & Austin, J. K. (1993). Causal attribution, perceived control, and adjustment in patients with lung cancer. *Oncology Nursing Forum, 20,* 23–30.

Bertero, C., Vanhanen, M., & Appelin, G. (2008). Receiving a diagnosis of inoperable lung cancer: Patients' perspectives of how it affects their life situation and quality of life. *Acta Oncologica, 47,* 862–869.

Chapple, A., Ziebland, S., & McPherson, A. (2004). Stigma, shame, and blame experienced by patients with lung cancer: Qualitative study. *British Medical Journal, 328,* 1470–1474.

Doka, K. (1997). When illness is prolonged: Implications for grief. In K. Doka & J. Davidson (Eds.), *Living with grief: When illness is prolonged* (pp. 5–16). Washington, DC: Taylor & Francis.

Doka, K. (2001). Grief, loss, and caregiving. In K. Doka & J. Davidson (Eds.), *Caregiving and loss: Family needs, professional responses* (pp. 215–230). Washington, DC: Hospice Foundation of America.

Doka, K. (Ed.). (2002). *Disenfranchised grief: New directions, challenges and strategies for practice.* Champaign, IL: Research Press.

Doka, K. (2005). Ethics, end-of-life decisions, and grief. In K. Doka (Ed.), *Living with grief: Ethical dilemmas at the end of life* (pp. 285–296). Washington, DC: Hospice Foundation of America.

Faller, H., Schilling, S., & Lang, H. (1995). Causal attributions and adaptation among lung cancer patients. *Journal of Psychosomatic Research, 39,* 619–627.

Figley, C. (Ed.). (1995). *Compassion fatigue: Coping with secondary stress disorder in those who treat the traumatized.* New York: Brunner/Mazel.

Fulton, R. (1987). The many faces of grief. *Death Studies, 11*(4), 243–256.

Humphrey, K. (2009). *Counseling strategies for loss and grief.* Alexandria, VA: American Counseling Association.

Kastenbaum, R. (1988). Vicarious grief as an intergenerational phenomenon. *Death Studies, 12,* 447–453.

Lazarus, R. J., & Folkman, S. (1984). *Stress, appraisal and coping.* New York: BasicBooks.

Lev, E. (1989). A nurse's perspective on disenfranchised grief. In K. Doka (Ed.), *Disenfranchised grief: Recognizing hidden sorrow* (pp. 286–299). New York: Lexington Press.

Martin, T. A., & Doka, K. J. (1999). *Men don't cry, women do: Transcending gender stereotypes of grief.* Philadelphia, PA: Brunner-Mazel.

McClement, S., Chochinov, H. M., Hack, T., Hassard, T., Kristjanson, L. J., & Harlos, M. (2007). Dignity therapy: Family members, perspectives. *Journal of Palliative Medicine, 10,* 1076–1108.

Mumma, C., & McCorkle, R. (1983). Causal attribution and life-threatening disease. *International Journal of Psychiatry in Medicine, 12,* 311–319.

Nehari, M., Grebler, D., & Toren, A. (2007). A voice unheard: Grandparents' grief over children who died of cancer. *Mortality, 12,* 66–78.

Papadatou, D. (2000). A proposed model of health professionals' grieving process. *Omega: The Journal of Death and Dying, 41,* 59–77.

Rando, T. A. (1983). An investigation into grief and adaptation in parents whose children have died from cancer. *Journal of Pediatric Psychology, 8,* 3–20.

Rando, T. A. (1993). *Treatment of complicated mourning.* Champaign, IL: Research Press.

Sanders, C. (1983). Effects of sudden vs. chronic illness on bereavement outcomes. *Omega: The Journal of Death and Dying, 13,* 227–241.

Tomarken, A., Holland, J., Schachter, S., Vanderwerker, L., Zuckerman, E., Nelson, C., et al. (2008). Factors of complicated grief pre-death in caregivers of cancer patients. *Psycho-Oncology, 17,* 105–111.

Vachon, M. (1987). *Occupational stress in the care of the critically ill, the dying, and the bereaved.* New York: Hemisphere.

Worden, J. W. (2009). *Grief counseling and grief therapy: A handbook of the mental health practitioner* (4th ed.). New York: Springer.

Personal Perspective: Antonia's Story

Yvette Colón

The hospice doctor and nurse were at my mother's bedside. I watched them give her information. Lots of it. They asked her to make decisions about medications. They encouraged her to make choices about the kind of care they were offering. I knew from experience that my mother, Antonia, didn't like making quick decisions about serious issues. I wanted to respect her right to make those decisions for herself and so I held back from interrupting. I sat by the foot of the bed, listening and watching. There was a pause in the conversation. My mother turned slightly away from the doctor and nurse and looked directly at me. She said nothing, but held my gaze for a long time. In that moment I knew that she trusted me completely. I knew she wanted me to help her make decisions about her care. She wanted help and guidance at the end of her life. Gathering all my knowledge as a clinical social worker and all my courage and love as a daughter, I outlined a short-term plan that was acceptable to everyone. Nine days later, my mother died.

It had all started just 3 weeks earlier. I always knew I would be called on to help my parents when they became ill and when they reached the end of their lives. It never occurred to me that I would be both blessed and burdened to be their social worker as well as their daughter. As a longtime clinical social worker, I have spent an entire career working with people with cancer and at the end of their lives. When I was diagnosed with ovarian cancer at the age of 27, I was working in a different field. My parents did not handle my diagnosis or treatment well; having a sick child, even one who was a young adult, was not the natural order of things. I got better and moved on with my life. It was only through my own experience and the profound influence of my support group social worker that I eventually returned to school to become an oncology social worker.

I remember the day as if it was yesterday. I was in Texas for a conference when I called my mom on a Wednesday to wish her a happy 74th birthday.

"Hi, Mom. Happy Birthday!" I said. She replied, "Oh, thank you. I guess I should tell you I'm having surgery on Friday." I was alarmed, "Surgery? Ma, what's going on? I talk to you all the time and you never mentioned surgery!" She was so matter of fact it could have been a comedy routine, but there was nothing funny about it. She plainly stated, "Oh, you're so busy. I didn't want to bother you." I hung up the phone, caught between the feelings that either something very bad was about to happen or that my mom was simply going in the hospital for a routine procedure.

My father faxed me my mother's medical information to my conference hotel with the hope that I could make some sense of it for him. I soon discovered that for months mom had been experiencing increasing pain and fatigue. She casually chalked it up to an exacerbation of a previous chronic pain condition, but decided she might as well have a full body scan. The doctor's report mentioned ascites and peritoneal carcinomatosis. My heart sank. My parents didn't know what that meant. I did. I immediately left the conference and flew to California to be with them. The diagnosis was grim: pancreatic cancer. There were lots of conversations and consultations—with her surgeon, the pathologist, with other family members who wanted to know what was going on and how to help. At first, the goal was to help mom recover from surgery, go home, and possibly have treatment as an outpatient. Mom was most concerned with being able to eat and keep up her strength. Before the week ended, she agreed to total parenteral nutrition, or TPN, which would provide all or most of her nutritional requirements intravenously. My father and I spent the next several days with her in the hospital, keeping her company, walking with her and watching television together.

It was almost like out of a textbook. One day in the hospital, my mom decided she wanted to go home. She knew she wasn't making much progress in her treatment of the disease, but she was reluctant to "give up" the TPN. Unfortunately, the TPN would make her care much more difficult outside of the hospital. We requested a second opinion about chemotherapy options from a medical oncologist. As fate would have it, he happened to be from the very medical center where I was treated 24 years earlier. He had a sensitive conversation with my mom and was frank about his belief that chemotherapy would not give her any more time. He was able to talk to her about the quality of her life and how he felt the chemotherapy would only erode it. He was kind to give her a prognosis, to help her understand the gravity of her illness. I knew what was coming: a prognosis of 6 to 9 months. Little did we know that it was only going to be less than 9 days. My mom courageously decided that she did not want to pursue chemotherapy treatment. "If it's not going to help me, I don't want it." After a week, my mom still was not ready to be discharged. I went home to Maryland to take care of some things, promising her I would return.

I called every day. First there was talk of discharge from the hospital, then there was none—only more confusion about the plan to get mom home. I was in constant contact with my professional network, calling a social work friend who worked at City of Hope to find out the best home care and hospice programs in Los Angeles. I called social work and nursing friends at Johns Hopkins Hospital who then tapped into their oncology colleagues' collective knowledge to get feedback about my mom's treatment options, current care, ideas about what to expect, and facilitating and translating massive amounts of information for my medically unsophisticated parents. I was rich in resources. I was blessed. All the information and support helped me focus on what my mom needed: her final wish to be respected. She needed to die at home.

Over the phone, my mother began telling me her discharge plans. They changed every day. First she was to go home. Then she was to remain in the hospital. Then she was being considered for a transfer to a transitional care unit. Her doctors would be away, my parents were told, so most community services would be closed for the July 4th weekend and hospice services would not be able to start until the holiday was over. Nothing could happen before then. The hospital care team members told her and my dad this several times. She was so disappointed. She longed for the familiar sounds and smells of my childhood home tucked away far from this hospital setting.

Not being able to be discharged until after the holiday weekend? That didn't sound right to me. I was concerned that if my mom went to transitional care, she would never be strong enough to go home. That was all she really wanted. From Maryland, I flew to California again and drove directly to the hospital to have a serious conversation with Mom about how she wanted to die. She decided that she would give up the TPN and go home with hospice care. On July 3, we all met early with the hospital's palliative care nurse to initiate the plan for discharge. After our meeting, a referral was made to hospice and we met with the intake nurse. In the course of their conversation, she asked Mom if she'd had a good life. Without hesitation, my mom said, "Oh yes. I've been very lucky. I've had a wonderful life." Afterwards, I left the hospital to clean the house and await delivery of a hospital bed and other medical equipment. My mother would be moving into my old room. My mom was discharged from the hospital, went home, and received her first visit from the hospice social worker and nurse on the Fourth of July. It was the birthday celebration of our country and the celebration of my mother being able to live out her life as she had always intended—in her home with her family by her side.

She sent my father and me to the cemetery to buy a burial plot in a place where other family members and friends were buried. She said, "When people come to visit me, they can visit them too." She asked us to return with a price list of other products and services at the funeral home. She wanted to make sure we didn't spend a lot of money. She outlined exactly what she wanted when the time came: a simple casket, a day of visitation, a Catholic mass and burial. She thoroughly enjoyed the Hispanic baby food we bought so that she could again experience some of the flavors and aromas of her Cuban childhood. She asked for specific visitors—her brother, nieces, other family members, and lifelong friends. She wanted them all to make special visits so that she could say goodbye to them. We all worked on a medication chart so that my 72-year-old father would know exactly what to give her at the right times. I went over the plan to call hospice and not 911 in case of an emergency.

My mom and I spent an afternoon with my laptop computer and her favorite CDs, copying the songs she wanted played at her service. We spent another lovely evening sitting together as a family watching the DVD of the 2006 Hospice Foundation of America Teleconference in which I was a panelist. She teased me about the new suit I wore, knowing that I had no interest in fashion and admittedly did not often dress myself without someone else's fashion advice. She wanted to know who had bought me that snazzy suit. I marveled at her resolve, even while I knew how difficult it really was for her, for me, for all of us.

Once my mother was settled at home I found myself leaving again. I had planned a vacation with my own family and my mom encouraged me to go. "You can always come back and see me after your vacation."

My vacation was anything but restful. I was constantly distracted by thoughts of my mom and her courage. I was clear across the country now, in rural Michigan where there was very patchy cell phone service. I tried to talk with her every day, but I couldn't receive calls as they came in. Instead, I would have to leave our lake cabin and drive into town a few times a day to retrieve my messages from the corner of the supermarket parking lot where the cell phone reception was the strongest. I was frantic. One morning the message was from the hospice social worker, expressing alarm at mom's quick decline. I had a long conversation with her and made quick plans to cut my vacation short and go back. I had only been in Michigan for 4 days. I was on my way to the local airport to fly to Los Angeles when my cell phone was active again and I listened to my messages. There was a simple one from my father. "Yvette, call home. Mom died this morning." He cried. That was the longest plane ride of my entire life.

When I got to the house, she was already gone. We drove immediately to the cemetery to buy the casket and make arrangements for the service and funeral. And even though my mom wanted us to be practical, we splurged on one thing we knew she would love: a polished oak casket with brass details.

There were many things I discovered during this short time at the end of my mother's life and beyond. She was realistic and humorous and surprisingly strong to the end. She had a strong faith in God, the depth of which I had never realized. She was profoundly appreciative of the care that my father gave her: "I never knew he loved me so much." When she came home from the hospital to find everything clean and neat and ready, she said to me, "I knew I could count on you." Two days before she died, she was teaching my cousins all about Medicare and Medigap so that they'd know how to choose the right coverage when they turn 65.

There were other things I acknowledged as I really looked at all the photos in my childhood home, ones I had only glanced at before and now I really saw them as they were meant to be seen. My parents were beautiful when they were young adults and starting on their life together; they were able to achieve so much with so few resources. They gave me so much without me ever really knowing how much it had cost them. They were terrific as their own individual people with dreams and aspirations. I recalled how much fun it was to cram so many people into small apartments for parties when I was a kid, when my family was so much larger than it is now and everyone was so cool and so happy.

I have also learned much more about my father since my mother died. When she was alive, I would call and if my dad answered, he'd say something like, "Did your mom tell you we got a new refrigerator? It was a big job to get it into the kitchen. Here she is. She wants to talk to you." And she and I would talk for an hour or more about who came to visit, who got married or divorced, where people went on vacation, who changed jobs or got in trouble at school. Now without her, I've learned that my dad is crazy about chocolate, that he loves Cirque du Soleil, that he has a great sense of humor and an easy-going personality. And I've learned exactly what he wants when it is his time to die.

My mother died exactly 1 month after her 74th birthday and only 28 days after the surgery that started this journey. The hospice care team, especially my mom's social worker and primary nurse, were wonderful and the program provided incredible support to both my parents. My father and I take great comfort in knowing that my mom got everything she wanted: to leave the hospital, to die at home, to go quickly, and to be pain-free. She was peaceful and comfortable when she died in her sleep.

My ability not only to find resources, but to activate them quickly, and to communicate with a far-flung network of oncology colleagues was the result of being a social worker. Everyone returned my calls quickly—the surgeon, the medical oncologist, nurses on the unit, professionals who were asked for favors by my friends. My boss and coworkers were very flexible and supportive. Everyone said we'd have to wait until the holiday was over and everyone was back at work, but I knew there were ways to overcome those barriers. My experience, however, is sadly not the norm for most patients and families who have to navigate through a complex, unknown healthcare maze. Most do not have a network of healthcare professionals who can offer advice, recommendations, and resources openly and directly. Ultimately, I've come to see the burden of being my mother's social worker as a blessing; and the privilege of being her daughter as a lifetime joy.

Yvette Colón, MSW, ACSW, BCD, is the director of education and Internet services at the American Pain Foundation. She is on the faculty at Smith College School for Social Work, and she has published and lectured extensively on end-of-life social work practice, pain management, psychosocial oncology, diversity, and technology-based social work services. Ms. Colón serves as co-coordinator of the Association of Oncology Social Work's Pain & Palliative Care Special Interest Group, an editorial board member of the Journal of Social Work *in end-of-life and palliative care, and a governing board member of the Intercultural Cancer Council. She is a member of the steering committee of the Emerging Network of Social Workers in End-of-Life and Palliative Care and recently served on the board of directors of the National Association of Social Workers. Ms. Colón holds a master's degree in social work from Smith College School for Social Work and is currently a PhD candidate in clinical social work at New York University.*

Index

A

Acetaminophen
  description and uses, 61

Adolescents. *See* Children and adolescents with cancer

Advance directives.
  description, 93–94, 113
  importance of, 113–114

AIDS and Its Metaphors (Sontag), 40

Alkylating chemotherapeutic agents, 57

American Academy of Pediatrics, 144

American Cancer Society
  Quality of Life Survey for Caregivers, 132–133
  Web site, 74

American Society for Control of Cancer, 6–7

Anthracyclines, 58

Anticipatory grief and anticipatory mourning
  accuracy of expectations and, 171–172
  advance planning of funeral or memorial services, 176–177
  anticipated losses, 171–172
  "disease" compared with "illness," 170
  forewarning and, 171
  grief reactions, 172–174
  "mourning" compared with "grief," 174
  mourning responses, 174–175
  opportunities for growth, 176–177
  phases of living with cancer, 170–171
  practical considerations, 176
  suggestions for family members and care providers, 178–179
  suggestions for individuals who are living with cancer, 177–178
  time with cancer as "pressured" and "precious," 176

Antimetabolites, 58

Antitumor antibiotics, 58

Aristotle
  "metaphor" definition, 42
  Poetics, 42

Art therapy
  children and adolescents with cancer and, 138–139, 143

Autonomy concept, 33–34, 88–89

B

Barnes, P. M.
  estimates of CAM use, 67

Beale, E. A.
  guideline for communicating with children and adolescents and their families about cancer treatment and dying, 140–141

Behavioral self-blame
  description, 126
  effect on psychological adjustment, 134

Beresford, B.
  unique psychosocial needs of adolescents with cancer, 141

Bingley, A. F.
  changes over time in the volume and location of narratives of illness, 48

Boston, P.
  culturally appropriate education efforts, 9

Brachytherapy, 59–60

Breast cancer
  advanced breast cancer as a chronic disease, 85
  history of smoking and, 131
  impact of self-blame and psychological adjustment, 125–126
  in men, 152, 153
  patients' uncertainty about the etiology of their cancer, 131
  practice focus, 153
  treatment of metastatic cancer, 84

Brescia, Dr. Michael
  process of metastasis, 110

Bulman, R. J.
  self-blame in coping with cancer causation, 125

C

CAM therapies. *See* Complementary and alternative medicine therapies

Cancer. *See also* End-stage cancer; *specific types of cancer*
  changes in the manifestations of, 41
  as a chronic illness, 22, 41, 83–87
  classification of, 1
  definition, 169
  estimated mortality rate, 1
  future considerations for patient care, 21–22
  journey metaphor, 46–49
  as a master illness, 41
  paternalism and self-determinism and, 47, 49

phases of living with cancer, 170–171
reluctance of oncologists to discuss prognosis, 46
significance of, 151–152
types and manifestations of, 169, 181
uncertainties about key processes, 41
warfare metaphor, 39–40, 41, 49, 86–87

Candib, L. M.
social structural factors in cancer, 158

Carcinomas, 1

Caregiver Guilt Scale, 133

Caregivers. *See also* Family caregivers; Formal caregivers
interventions after a cancer death, 185–187
isolation of, 184
role as a complicating factor in grief, 184–185
role as a facilitating factor in grief, 184
stress issues, 184–185
suggestions for family members and care providers,
178–179

Case studies, 17, 26, 28–29, 31, 33, 35, 112, 113–114,
115, 116, 117–118, 118–119

Cassileth, B. R.
estimates of CAM use among adult cancer patients,
67–68

Center for Mind-Body Medicine
training for "integrative-care counselors" for CAM
therapies, 74–75

Cervical cancer
patients' perceptions of factors causing, 127–129

Characterological self-blame
description, 126
effect on psychological adjustment, 134

Chemotherapy
as adjuvant therapy, 6
administration routes, 57
agents for, 57–58
decision-making issues, 27–29
"doing something" concept and, 99
growth of options for, 84
historical background, 6
limitations of statistics for decision making about,
30–31
long-term oral therapies, 84–85
mechanism of action, 57
objective of, 6
Saul case example, 31, 33, 35
side effects, 57
uses for, 57

Children and adolescents with cancer
art therapy and, 138–139
death of a child as a complicating factor in grief, 185
estimated number of children diagnosed with cancer
each year, 137
exploring death-related questions, 140–141
guidelines for communication, 140–141
imparting information about their illness, 139–141
importance of trust, 139–140
Internet use and, 141–142

personal perspective: Vivienne's story, 147–150
support staff role, 138
transition to palliative care, 137, 143–144
trends in cancer deaths for adolescents ages 15–19, 137
unique needs of adolescents, 141–142

Clayton, J. M.
fostering coping skills and nurturing hope while
discussing poor prognoses with patients, 104

Clinical trials
ethical issues, 87–88

Clow, B.
shunning the diagnosis of cancer, 43

Cochrane Library
Cochrane Reviews, 73
peer-reviewed studies of CAM therapies, 73

Codeine
moderate pain treatment, 61

Coles, Robert
art therapy for children and adolescents with cancer,
139, 143

Communication issues
challenges in discussing poor prognoses, 100, 110–111
physician-patient therapeutic communication, 73
protocols for communicating terminal prognoses,
100–102

The Compassionate Friends, 166

Complementary and alternative medicine therapies
adding questions about CAM on patient health
assessment forms, 75
danger of using CAM without discussing the use with
healthcare practitioners, 70
description, 68
estimates of CAM use, 67
importance of patient-physician communication, 68,
70–71, 75
major domains of, 68
nursing and medical school curricula and, 71, 73
patient reluctance to report use of to healthcare
practitioners, 70–71
popularity of, 67
reasons why patients do not discuss their use of CAM
therapies with their healthcare practitioners, 70–71
reasons why patients use CAM therapies, 69–70
relief of chemotherapy-related side effects and, 69–70
resources for, 73–74
responsibilities of healthcare practitioners, 72–73

Complicating factors in cancer deaths
blame, guilt, and disenfranchised grief, 182–183
caregivers' experience, 184–185
death of a child, 185
ethical decisions at the end of life, 183–184
formal caregivers and, 190
perception that the patient didn't fight hard enough to
survive, 183
personality changes, 181, 182
physical disfigurement, 181–182
prolonged illness and grief, 181–182

Congestive heart failure
John case example, 17
needs of patients with, 19–20

Continuing Bonds model of grief
metaphors of illness and, 46

Coping skills
after a cancer death, 188

Correa-Velez, I.
questions to ask patients about CAM therapies, 75
reasons why patients use CAM therapies, 69

Corticosteroids, 58

Costanzo, E. S.
patients' perceptions of factors causing their cancers, 127–128
positive attitude as a factor in preventing cancer recurrence, 128

Christakis, N.
"prophecy effect" of prognoses by oncologists, 47

Cultural issues
culturally appropriate education efforts, 9
fear of cancer, 9–10
prevalence of cancer in industrialized countries, 3–4, 9
stigma of cancer, 10

D

Damasio, Antonio
physicians' awareness of their own feelings, 100

Dana-Farber Cancer Institute
percentage of breast cancer affecting men, 152

Dartmouth Institute for Health Policy and Clinical Practice
benefits of more medical care for chronically ill patients, 32

Decision-making issues
determining code status, 34
forgoing further treatment, 83–84, 90, 93
Jessie case example, 26
life-threatening diagnosis, 25–36
limitations of quantitative methods, 29–31
paradoxes, 31–35
personal growth, 35–36
quality of life, 26, 28–29
using narrative for decision making, 27–29

Dementia
future considerations for patient care, 21–22
hospice needs for patients with, 16, 17, 20, 21

Dignity therapy
description, 186

Doka, K. J.
concerns of living with a life-threatening illness, 114
gendered patterns of grieving, 154, 156
phases of living with cancer, 170–171

Dual Process Model of grief
metaphors of illness and, 46

Dunn, Hank
challenges of siblings when they have to make end-of-life decisions for their parents, 113

E

Ebers papyrus, 3

Education for Physicians on End-of-Life Care
protocol for delivering bad news, 102

Edwin Smith papyrus, 3, 5

Eisenberg, D. M.
description of CAM therapies, 68
estimates of CAM use, 67
integration of CAM therapy information into medical education curricula, 73, 75
physician discussions of CAM therapies with patients, 71

Elderly persons
hospice needs for patients with dementia, 16, 17, 20, 21

Elliot, J.
reasons why patients use CAM therapies, 69

Emotions
after a cancer death, 187
gender relationship with, 152
role in the transition to palliative care, 99–100

End-of-life care
aggressive treatment to prolong life and, 97–98
challenges of discussing terminal diagnoses with patients and their families, 101–102
compared with palliative care, 56
complicating factors, 183–184
conflicts between family members, 183
ethical issues, 112–114, 183–184
percentage of all Medicare spending in the last year of patients' lives, 97

End-stage cancer
case studies, 112, 113–114, 115, 116, 117–118, 118–119
challenges in making the decision to forgo curative therapy, 109
ethical issues and concerns, 112–114
life-threatening illness as a family illness, 110, 163
medical issues and concerns, 110–112
psychological issues and concerns, 116–119
spiritual/existential issues and concerns, 114–116

Endometrial cancer
patients' perceptions of factors causing, 127–129

Ernst, E.
estimates of CAM use among adult cancer patients, 67–68

Ethical issues
advance-care planning, 93–94, 113–114
benefits and burdens of continuing treatment near the end of life, 93–94
benefits of newer treatments, 83

cancer survivorship, 86–87
clinical trials and novel therapies, 87–88
cost of newer treatments, 83, 85, 90
deciding to forgo further treatment, 83–84, 90, 93
end-of-life care, 112–114, 183–184
goals of treatment and goals of care, 91–92, 113
health care practitioners' discussions about CAM
    therapy use with patients, 72
long-term oral therapies, 84–85
managing cancer as a chronic disease, 83–86
open access to hospice care, 90–91
pain relief for dying patients, 63
physician-patient collaboration, 94–95
shared decision-making paradigm, 85–86
"therapeutic misconception," 87–88, 89
weighing benefits and burdens of treatment, 88–90

Ethical wills, 114, 186

F

Family caregivers
    "caregiver" definition, 132
    Caregiver Guilt Scale, 133
    feelings of guilt among, 132–134
    suggestions for family members and care providers,
        178–179

Formal caregivers. See also Healthcare practitioners
    grief issues after a cancer death, 189–191

Foucault, Michel
    archaeology of medicine, 42–43

Fouladbakhsh, J.
    estimates of CAM use, 68

Frank, Arthur
    distinction between "disease" and "illness," 170
    illness as an opportunity, 175
    narratives of illness, 48–49

Frankl, Viktor
    loss of meaning in one's life as the cause of human
        suffering, 115

Fried, T. R.
    percentage of people whose physicians had told them
        their disease was fatal, 102

Froggatt, K.
    nurses and metaphors of illness, 45

Fulton, R.
    Stockholm syndrome and the health professional-
        patient relationship, 189–190

G

Galen
    belief that cancer was incurable, 5
    "oncos" term for cancer, 3
    tumor removal and, 5

Gender factors in cancer
    gender differences in reactions to the cancer of one's
        parents, 154, 156
    gender relationship with emotion, 152
    healthy lifestyle, 154
    help-seeking behavior, 154
    impact on identity, 157–158
    impact on specific stakeholders, 159
    influence one partner has on the other's adjustment,
        157
    organizational and other contextual factors, 156
    practice focuses, 153, 155
    significance of cancer, 151–152
    significance of gender, 152–157
    society's expectations of men and, 154

Genomics
    description, 27

Gibbs, R. W., Jr.
    metaphors used by cancer patients, 47, 48

Gordon, J.
    health care practitioners as "healing partners," 75

Grant, Pres. Ulysses S.
    cancer battle, 4

Gray, R.
    reluctance of physicians to discuss CAM therapy use
        with patients, 71

Grief
    as an inherent part of the cancer experience, 192
    definition, 169, 172
    "mourning" compared with, 174

Grief after a death from cancer
    complicating factors in cancer deaths, 181–185
    interventions, 185–191

Grief and cancer
    anticipatory grief and anticipatory mourning, 169–179
    central concepts, 169
    chapter overview, 163–164
    gendered patterns of grieving, 154, 156
    grief after a death from cancer, 181–192
    meaning reconstruction and, 156–157
    personal perspective: Antonia's story, 195–200
    personal perspective: he was still our child, 165–167

Grief reactions
    appropriateness of, 173
    categories of, 173
    individual nature of, 174
    social dimensions, 173
    spiritual dimensions, 173

Gross, C. P.
    disparities in cancer morbidity, 124

Guilt and self-blame in coping with cancer causation. See
    also Stigma of cancer
    blame, guilt, and disenfranchised grief as complicating
        factors in cancer deaths, 182–183
    breast cancer and, 125–126
    family caregivers and guilt, 132–134
    guilt after the cancer patient dies, 182
    gynecological cancer and, 127–129
    head and neck cancers and, 132
    importance of the issue, 125

interaction between attributing cancer to an unhealthy lifestyle and dietary change in predicting anxiety (figure), 129

lung cancer and perceived risk among smokers, 129–132

significantly different mean scores of Perceived Cancer-Related Stigma items at enrollment (table), 127

Gynecological cancer. *See also* Cervical cancer; Endometrial cancer; Ovarian cancer

interaction between attributing cancer to an unhealthy lifestyle and dietary change in predicting anxiety (figure), 129

lifestyle issues, 128–129

significantly different mean scores of Perceived Cancer-Related Stigma items at enrollment (table), 127

H

HAART. *See* Highly active antiretroviral therapies

Hawkins, A. H.

"pathographies" of cancer patients, 43

Head and neck cancers

guilt and self-blame issues in causation of, 132

Health care practitioners. *See also* Formal caregivers

adding questions about CAM on patient health assessment forms, 75

CAM therapy responsibilities, 72–73

challenges of discussing terminal diagnoses with patients and their families, 101–102

continuing education opportunities in CAM therapy, 73

discussing the use of CAM therapies with patients, 68, 70

grief issues after a cancer death, 189–191

need for greater awareness of the reasons why patients use CAM therapies, 70

physicians' modification of information given to patients when they think that the truth will have a bad outcome, 110

reasons why HCPs don't ask patients about CAM therapy use, 71–72

role of emotion in treating patients at the end of life, 99–100

therapeutic communication with patients, 73

Highly active antiretroviral therapies, 15, 16

Hill, Dr. John

snuffing tobacco and nose cancers, 8

Hinds, P. S.

end-of-life decision making for parents of children and adolescents with cancer, 137

Hippocrates

belief that cancer was incurable, 5

"carcinoma" term for cancer, 3

humoral theory of health and illness, 4

Historical background

cancer terminology, 3

causes of cancer, 4–5

hospice care, 13–17

prevention of cancer, 8

treatment of cancer, 5–8

"war on cancer," 7

HIV/AIDS

highly active antiretroviral therapies and, 15, 16

hospice care role, 15–16

Hockey, J.

clergy's metaphor of the body as a container, 45

Hoffman, R.

significance of gender in cancer, 159

Hospice care

decline in proportion of U.S. hospice cancer admissions 2000-2007 (figure), 19

decrease in the number of patients with cancer, 18

end-stage cancer and, 109–119

estimated percentage of patients needing, 16

family and patient as the unit of care, 15

future considerations for, 21–22

growth in live discharges U.S. hospices 2002-2007 (figure), 20

historical background, 13–17

HIV/AIDS and, 15–16

interdisciplinary approach, 14

late patient admission into, 111

median length of stay in a hospice program, 109

model for, 14–15

need for care in the home, 15

need to preserve hope and, 110

open access movement, 90–91

palliative care and, 56

six-month prognosis and, 15, 111

survival time for hospice patients with lung cancer, 98

trajectories of death and, 16–17

Hoxsey, Harry

cancer treatment, 7–8

Human genome project

contribution to the understanding of cancer, 9

Hydromorphone

dosage intervals and, 64

moderate pain treatment, 61

I

Illness as Metaphor (Sontag), 39–41, 43–44, 46, 49, 175

Internet

adolescents with cancer and, 141–142

parents use of for information, 142

Interventions after a cancer death

after the death, 187–189

as the patient approaches death, 185–186

when death occurs, 186–187

Irish Sisters of Charity

Our Lady's Hospice founding, 13

J

Jackson, V. A.
  emotions of oncologists, 100

Jansen, S. J. T.
  percentage of breast cancer patients on chemotherapy
    who would continue on it even if there was no
    clinical benefit, 99

Journey metaphors for cancer, 47, 49

K

Kastenbaum, R.
  "vicarious grief" description, 164

Kelly, Orville
  "make today count" concept, 175

Kennedy, Sen. Edward
  21st Century Cancer Access to Life-Saving Early
    Detection, Research, and Treatment (ALERT) Act
    sponsor, 7

Kirmayer, L.
  metaphors of illness, 47–48

Koch, Dr. William
  cancer treatment, 7

Krebiozen vaccine, 8

L

Lattanzi-Licht, M. E.
  society's expectations of men, 154

Lawton, J.
  gender identity and cancer, 158

Leukemias
  as chronic diseases, 85
  description, 1
  John case example, 28–29, 33, 35
  long-term oral therapy for chronic myelogenous
    leukemia, 84

Lifestyle issues
  gynecological cancer and, 128–129
  non-small-cell lung cancer and, 131–132

Little, Clarence Cook
  American Society for Control of Cancer leadership, 6

Little, M.
  gender identity and cancer, 158

Living eulogies, 186

Living wills. See Advance directives

LoConte, N. K.
  Perceived Cancer-Related Stigma scale, 127, 132

Lung cancer
  benefits of intensive care near the end of life, 98
  Jessie case example, 26
  non-small-cell lung cancer compared with other
    cancers, 130–132
  perceived risk among smokers, 129–130, 181, 182
  stigma of, 10, 130–132, 181, 182
  whole-brain radiation therapy, 59

Lymphomas
  as chronic diseases, 85
  description, 1

M

Mackillop, W. J.
  physicians' ability to predict survival rates for patients,
    111

Marshall, P. A.
  self-determinism of patients, 47
  therapeutic communication with patients, 73

Martin, T. L.
  gendered patterns of grieving, 154, 156

Master illnesses
  cancer as, 41
  description, 41
  postmodernism and, 41–42

M.D. Anderson Cancer Center
  description of CAM therapies, 68

Medicaid
  six-month prognosis and, 18, 20

*Medical Guidelines for Determining Prognosis in Selected
  Non-Cancer Diseases*, 17–18

Medicare
  percentage of all Medicare spending in the last year of
    patients' lives, 97
  six-month prognosis and, 18

Metaphors of illness
  contemporary, 44–49
  master illnesses, 41–42
  metaphor definitions, 42–43
  models of grief and, 46
  Susan Sontag's work, 39–41, 43–44, 46, 49, 175
  varieties of metaphor, 43–44

Methadone
  mechanism of action, 64
  moderate pain treatment, 61

Minimally invasive surgery
  description, 56

Mitotic inhibitors, 58

Miyaji, N.
  physicians' modification of information given to
    patients when they think that the truth will have a
    bad outcome, 110

Molecular genetics, 27

Morphine
  complications from, 63
  dosage and timing considerations, 62

moderate pain treatment, 61
onset of pain relief, 62
opioid rotation and, 63
severe pain treatment, 63
side effects, 63
upward dose titration, 62–63

Morphine sulfate instant-release
"breakthrough pain" and, 62
conversion to, 62
description and uses, 62
dosage considerations, 62

Mourning
anticipatory mourning focus, 175
compared with "grief," 174
complementary forms of, 174
definition, 169
post-death mourning focus, 175

N

Narratives of illness
decision-making issues, 27–29
description, 28
increase in the public domain, 48
types of, 48–49

National Cancer Act
provisions, 7

National Cancer Institute
autonomy of, 7
clinical trial registry, 87
establishment of, 6
Web site, 74

National Cancer Intelligence Network
men and healthy lifestyle, 154

National Center for Complementary and Alternative
Medicine
CAM therapies information, 74
fact sheets, 73–74
major domains of CAM therapies, 68
reviews of studies of efficacy, end points, and side
effects of CAM therapy, 72
use of CAM as complementary/integrative medicine,
76
Web site, 68, 74

National Hospice and Palliative Care Organization.
hospice needs for patients with solid organ failure and
dementia, 17
*Medical Guidelines for Determining Prognosis in
Selected Non-Cancer Diseases*, 17–18

National Institutes of Health Consensus Conference
efficacy of acupuncture in relieving chemotherapy-
related nausea and vomiting, 69

Nature of cancer
cultural perspective, 9–10
decision making, 25–36
historical perspective, 3–8, 9–10
history of hospice and, 13–22

metaphors of illness, 39–49
overview of chapters, 1–2

Neck cancers. *See* Head and neck cancers

Nerve blocks
severe pain treatment, 63

Neuropathic pain
description, 61
methadone treatment, 64

NHPCO. *See* National Hospice and Palliative Care
Organization

Nixon, Pres. Richard H.
"war on cancer," 7

Noncancer patients
care management for, 20
challenges of discharging from hospice care, 20–21
dementia patients, 20, 21
future considerations for patient care, 21–22
increase in hospice care for, 19–20
policy challenges in care for, 20–21
psychosocial concerns, 21

Nonsteroidal antiinflammatory drugs, 61

Nurses. *See* Formal caregivers; Health care practitioners

O

Opioids
moderate pain treatment, 61–64
use with cancer patients, 14

Our Lady's Hospice
founding of, 13

Ovarian cancer
difficulty of diagnosing, 154

Oxycodone
dosage considerations, 64
moderate pain treatment, 61

P

Paget, Stephen
metastasis process, 5

Palliative care. *See also* Transition to palliative care
categories of cancer pain, 61
children and adolescents and, 137, 139, 143–144
end-stage cancer and, 109–119
importance of, 55–56
need to preserve hope and, 110
WHO definition, 60

Palliative radiation
description and uses, 59

Palliative surgery
description, 56

Papadatou, D.
grief issues for healthcare professionals after a cancer
death, 190, 191

Paradoxes in decision making
  autonomy concept, 33–34
  definition, 32
  expecting the best, preparing for everything, 34–35
  mortality as a part of life, 32
  uncertainty about the future as a source of hope and
    anxiety, 33

Parker, P. A.
  qualities patients want in their oncologists, 99

Patenaude, A. F.
  gender differences in reactions to the cancer of one's
    parents, 154, 156

Perceived Cancer-Related Stigma scale
  guilt and self-blame assessment, 127, 132

Personal perspectives
  Antonia's story, 195–200
  He was still our child, 165–167
  Vivienne's story, 147–150

Physicians. See Formal caregivers; Health care
practitioners

Pitceathly, C.
  gender factors in cancer, 157

Platinum-based chemotherapeutic agents, 58

Poetics (Aristotle), 42

Pollack, K. I.
  "empathic opportunities" for oncologists, 100

Pott, Dr. Percival
  scrotum cancer in chimney sweeps, 8

Prevention efforts
  epidemiological study implications, 8
  historical background, 8

Prognostication
  improvement in accuracy for nonmalignant disease
    diagnoses, 17–18
  six-month prognosis and hospice eligibility, 15, 17–18

Prostate cancer
  brachytherapy, 59
  gender challenges, 154, 155
  history of smoking and, 131
  number of men diagnosed with annually, 152, 154
  patients' uncertainty about the etiology of their cancer,
    131
  practice focus, 155
  treatment options, 55
  "watchful waiting" and, 169

Psychological issues
  anxiety at the end of life, 118
  end-stage cancer and, 116–119
  feelings of helplessness, 118
  need to preserve autonomy, 118
  suicide risk, 116–118

Psychosocial aspects of cancer care
  chapter overview, 123–124
  children and adolescents with cancer, 123–124

  gender, 151–159
  guilt and self-blame in coping with cancer causation,
    125–134
  importance of treating the whole person, 123

Q

Quality of Life Survey for Caregivers
  description, 132–133

Quantitative methods
  description, 30
  limitations of in decision making, 29–31

R

Radiation therapy. See also X-rays
  brachytherapy, 59–60
  cancer confined to one area and, 59
  high-energy photon beams, 59
  palliative, 59

Ramazzini, Bernardino
  cervical cancer research, 8

Rand vaccine, 8

Reconstructive surgery, 56

Reichner, C. A.
  benefits of intensive care near the end of life for lung
    cancer patients, 98

Rhodes, C.
  gender identity and cancer, 157

Ricoeur, P.
  "metaphor" definition, 42

Rituals
  healing rituals, 115–116
  therapeutic, after a cancer death, 189

Roentgen, Wilhelm
  X-ray technology research, 5–6

Rolland, John S.
  family adaptation to cancer in children and
    adolescents, 142

Romero, C.
  self-forgiveness and spirituality as predictors of less
    mood disturbance and better quality of life for
    breast cancer patients, 126

S

Sarbin, T. R.
  dramaturgical or dramatistic social roles, 44

Sarcomas, 1

Saunders, Dr. Cicely
  hospice care development, 13, 14, 109

Schofield, P.
  facilitating the transition from curative to palliative
    care, 102

Self-blame. *See* Guilt and self-blame in coping with cancer causation

Sharma, G.
costs of care for ICU-admitted patients with lung cancer, 98

Six-month prognosis
hospice eligibility and, 15, 17–18, 20, 111
Medicare and Medicaid and, 18

Smith, L. K.
men's reluctance to seek help, 154

Smoking. *See* Tobacco use

Solid organ failure
future considerations for patient care, 21–22
hospice needs for patients, 16, 17, 19–20
John case example, 17

Somatic pain, 61

Sontag, Susan
AIDS and Its Metaphors, 40
Illness as Metaphor, 39–41, 43–44, 46, 49, 175

Sorkin, R. D.
evolutionary control mechanisms and the origins of cancer, 3

Sourkes, Barbara
Countertransference in Psychotherapy with Children and Adolescents, 138

Spall, B.
nurses and metaphors of illness, 45–46

Spillers, R. L.
caregiver guilt, 133–134

Spiritual/existential issues
end-stage cancer and, 114–116
healing rituals, 115–116

St. Christopher's Hospice, Sydenham, England
description, 13, 109

Stacey, J.
gender identity and cancer, 157

State Shame and Guilt Scale
guilt and self-blame assessment, 132

Stigma of cancer. *See also* Guilt and self-blame in coping with cancer causation
cultural issues, 10
lung cancer patients, 10, 130–132, 181, 182

Support groups, 189

SUPPORT study, 111

Surgery
historical background of surgical treatment of cancer, 5
overview of methods and uses, 56
prostate cancer treatment, 55

Surgical biopsies
description, 56

Surgical debulking
description, 56

Surgical staging
description, 56

T

Target Ovarian Cancer
difficulty of diagnosing ovarian cancer, 154

Target therapy, 60

Therapeutic misconception
description and ethical issues, 87–88
weighing benefits and burdens of treatment, 89

Tobacco use
head and neck cancers and, 132
perceived risk of lung cancer among smokers, 129–130, 181

Topoisomerase I and II inhibitors, 58

Transition to palliative care
agreeing to withdrawal of treatment and, 98–99
balancing realism and hope, 104
benefits of treatment to prolong life, 97–98
challenges of, 97–98
children and adolescents and, 137, 143–144
communication issues, 101–102
discussing the transition, 102–104
helpful interventions, 103–104
pain as the most common trigger for referral to, 102
role of emotion, 99–100

Treatment options. *See also specific treatments*
chemotherapy, 57–58
complementary and alternative medicine therapies, 67–76
cost of newer treatments, 83, 85, 90
ethical issues, 83–95
factors in, 169
historical background, 5–8
learning curve for patients and families, 27
modalities, 55
overview of chapters, 53–54
palliative care, 55–56, 60–64, 97–104
quackery and, 7–8
radiation therapy, 59–60
range of, 55–64
research on, 6–7
role of palliative care and hospice in end-stage cancer, 109–119
surgery, 56
targeted therapy, 60
21st Century Cancer Access to Life-Saving Early Detection, Research, and Treatment (ALERT) Act, 7

U

United Kingdom
   hospice care model, 14–15

U.S. Food and Drug Administration
   addictive potential of weak opioids, 61

V

Vachon, M.
   factors influencing adjustment to the death of a
      patient, 191

Virchow, Rudolph
   cancer cell derivation theory, 4

Visceral pain, 61

W

Wang, S.
   nurses' response to CAM therapy use by patients,
      71–72

Warfare metaphor for cancer, 39–40, 41, 49

Weigner, W.
   review of the safety and efficacy of CAM therapies, 74

Wetzel, M.
   integration of CAM therapy information into medical
      education curricula, 73, 75

Worden, J. W.
   categories of grief reactions, 173
   "mourning" compared with "grief," 174

World Health Organization
   analgesic ladder, 61
   environmental carcinogens, 8
   palliative care definition, 60

Wynia, M.
   physician discussions of CAM therapies with patients,
      71

X

X-rays. *See also* Radiation therapy
   historical background of use for diagnosis and
      treatment of cancer, 5–6

Z

Zhang, B.
   communication on end-of-life issues, 101

This book was produced as part of Hospice Foundation of America's annual *Living with Grief®* teleconference, a live educational program for professionals and students of end-of-life care. The topic for the 2010 teleconference was *Cancer and End-of-Life Care.* A DVD of the live program can be ordered by visiting www.hospicefoundation.org or calling 1-800-854-3402.